SCHAUMBURG TOWNSHIP

P9-DHK-712

3 1257 01956 7998

WITHDRAWN

Schaumburg Township District Library
130 South Roselle Road
Schaumburg, Illinois 60193

dream

NEW DREAMS

dream

NEW DREAMS

Reimagining My Life After Loss

JAI PAUSCH

CROWN ARCHETYPE

New York

Schaumburg Township District Library
130 South Roselle Road
Schaumburg, IL 60193

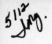

921
PAUSCH, J

3 1257 01956 7998

Copyright © 2012 by Elizabeth Jai Pausch
All rights reserved.

Published in the United States by Crown Archetype,
an imprint of the Crown Publishing Group,
a division of Random House, Inc., New York.

www.crownpublishing.com
Crown Archetype with colophon is a trademark of Random House, Inc.

Library of Congress Cataloging-in-Publication Data
Pausch, Jai, 1966–
  Dream new dreams : reimagining my life after loss / Jai Pausch. —1st ed.
    p. cm.
1. Pausch, Jai, 1966– 2. Women caregivers—United States—Biography. 3. Pancreas—
Cancer—Patients—Family relationships—United States. 4. Pausch, Randy—Health.
5. Death—Psychological aspects. I. Title.
  RC280.P25P38 2012
  616.994370092—dc23
  [B]
                           2011046264

ISBN 978-0-307-88850-1
eISBN 978-0-307-88852-5

Printed in the United States of America

Book design by Ralph Fowler
Jacket design by Michael Nagin
Hand lettering on jacket by Mary Ciccotto

10   9   8   7   6   5   4   3   2   1

FIRST EDITION

To all the people

who care for ill and dying loved ones

and who struggle to do the best they can

without the proper training and resources to help them

CONTENTS

FOREWORD

In 2008 my husband died after a two-year battle with pancreatic cancer. While he received the best medical care possible, from the time he was diagnosed in 2006 until his death, I was his primary caregiver. In spring 2009, I participated in an event sponsored by my local Jewish Community Center (JCC) called the Week of the Caregiver. It was my first time speaking about my experience. In putting together my talk, I had to force myself to examine the struggles I had faced over the previous couple of years. First, I had to convince myself that my voice and perspective were valuable. Then I had to pull together my hard-won lessons, striving to take the ugly, nasty things I had been through and do some good with them; to spin some straw into gold so to speak, and to share them with others who were walking or might walk the same path. I was reassured to see that what I had to say struck a chord. The hundred people in the audience not only listened attentively, but some also took notes.

After the talk, I shook hands and listened as people shared their own experiences. Their grief and the guilt they felt for mistakes they perceived they had made echoed some of my own feelings. I asked myself, Where is the help for folks like us who tirelessly give to our dying loved one? Why wasn't the medical community concerned about the people who struggle to carry the medical burden while also meeting normal everyday demands? I wanted to hug them all and wipe away their self-doubts and replace it with self-forgiveness. I wished for a magic wand to create a support network at every oncology clinic for the caregiver whom the medical community assumes can and will manage complicated medical care while grappling with their own complicated and sometimes overwhelming emotions. Though I did achieve my initial goal, I walked away feeling like there was so much more that needed to be done.

Over the next two years, I had other opportunities to talk about the impact cancer has had on my life and on my family. Each time I spoke to a group or met with a cancer-related medical professional, I brought the caregiver's role and needs to their attention. I wanted to shine a spotlight on the person in the treatment room who is so often overlooked, along with his or her needs and abilities. Although I couldn't travel and give talks and advocate for the caregiver's silent plight, I thought a book could reach so many more people.

I wanted my story to be useful to others, not a tell-all about the professor who wrote *The Last Lecture*. I started by using my JCC talk as the basic framework for my narrative and explored the unique challenges and complex issues I had faced as a caregiver. I spoke with grief counselors and palliative care doctors and met with dozens of caregivers for both cancer and Alzheimer's patients. Although each person's experience is unique, the overarching struggles are universal. Mining my own experiences forced me to dig into a wound still raw and painful, which had both positive and negative effects on me.

On the upside, writing has been a tremendous aid in helping me to heal myself; the process allowed me to see my strength and resilience. I've been able to move forward in a new direction for myself and my family. It's also given me the opportunity to come to peace with a lot of bad stuff that happened.

On the down side, I'm not able to put my past behind me completely. My years with Randy get brought up in some way, shape, or form every day. It could be an e-mail from a pancreatic cancer advocacy group or someone recognizing my name that resurrects my past. Three and a half years after Randy's death I still suffer from nightmares, talking in my sleep as my subconscious relives the most traumatic moments during that very trying time in my life. My new husband, Rich, wakes me from my nightmares, quiets my sleep talk, and soothes me back to sleep. It's not the way I wanted to start a new chapter in my life. It's not the happy Hollywood ending I was hoping for, but I know my story doesn't end with this book.

Ultimately, my dream is that my story will legitimize what caregivers undergo willingly and bravely as they care for a person they love. Patients need and deserve support, but it's time for us as a community to understand the suffering that is shouldered, sometimes silently, by our family members, neighbors, friends, and coworkers. We need to offer help to these people, to develop and implement programs at cancer centers and other organizations. We need to empathize with that person taking on the duty of overseeing the patient's care and well-being. Finally, we need to care for the caregiver.

1

Living the Dream

S O I CAN PICK UP the block and throw it?" Randy asked incredulously. He was learning about computer graphic research at the University of North Carolina, where I was working while studying for my PhD exams in comparative literature. Randy was a computer science professor at Carnegie Mellon University in Pittsburgh researching virtual reality and human-computer interaction. Standing in the virtual reality lab, he looked like a thirty-seven-year-old kid playing a Wii video game, game controller in hand. Instead of viewing the computer-generated world on a television mounted on a wall, he was looking at a screen inside a specialized helmet. Nowadays, many Americans are familiar with holding a device to make objects or avatars move within a video game. But fourteen years ago, this technology was not yet mainstream, nor was it a game; rather it was an experiment to see how compelling virtual reality could be. In this demonstration, throwing the block was not part of the program's functions, but Randy didn't know that, and he was asking a million questions. I had noticed his inquisitiveness earlier in the morning as we toured other parts of the virtual reality lab. Walking beside him, I could tell he was genuinely interested in our research, soaking it all in. It was obvious to me he was smart. What else would you expect of a Carnegie Mellon professor? But Randy was surprisingly down-to-earth. When I had first met him that morning, and in previous e-mails, he insisted I call him Randy, not Dr. Pausch. He had no need to stand on ceremony or demand acknowledgment of his title, which was a very refreshing change from the norm in academia. I felt instantly comfortable with him even after having only just met him. And I wanted to get to know him better.

I was taken with his easygoing and playful nature. I guess that's why I tricked him. "Oh, yes, you can throw the block into the next room"—I lied when Randy was trying out the pit demonstration. So he picked up the block with the game controller, raised it over his head and gave it a good toss. "It didn't work!" he exclaimed. "Well, you must have released the button too soon," I said. I looked around at the graduate students who were running the research demonstration. We smiled and laughed a little, all in on the joke. Randy tried several times to pick up and throw the block until he must have heard us laughing. Then he lifted up the helmet, looked at me with a twinkle in his eyes and laughed along with us. It was love at first sight between us. I could see this six-foot-tall, thick-dark-haired, smart man who had a great sense of humor and was so secure with himself. He must have thought I was attractive and maybe a little bewitching because he asked me to meet him that night. Of course, I was thrilled and accepted his invitation. I literally sat by the phone waiting for him to call after his dinner meeting. As the time of his expected call came and went, I figured he had changed his mind, that I had been imagining the connection I had felt with him earlier in the day, that I had fooled myself into believing his intentions were serious. Then the phone rang. Randy apologized for calling me after he said he would, but the meeting had run late. He really wanted to meet me and hoped it wasn't too late. I picked up my purse and headed out the door with my heart pounding.

It's bittersweet for me to think about how we first met and started dating, how I came to trust him and believe in him enough to try marriage one more time. I had had a rocky first marriage to my college sweetheart, which left me cynical about marriage and my ability to find a man who could stay true to those timeless wedding vows to love, honor, and cherish. Looking back on those first days and weeks pains me so much. It tears open the wound that has only begun to heal. It hurts to think about that first date when we walked along Franklin Street in Chapel Hill and held hands. I had to reach for his hand to hold him back a little, to keep pace with him, because he was such a fast walker and I was much slower. I remember how soft his hands were, how hairy his knuckles were, and that he bit his fingernails just like me. When we held hands, he would sometimes rub my fingers close to the knuckle, which melted away all my stress and left me boneless. It wasn't a "yin and yang" attraction. It was that we somehow fit together—intellectually, playfully, and emotionally.

He was in Chapel Hill for only a couple of days, and his time was booked for meetings with university faculty. But on the second day of his visit, Randy asked if I would like him to stay another day so we could go out again. I was flattered and said yes. After I got off from work, he rode the public bus with me back to my apartment. He lost no time in changing his schedule, making phone calls on his cell phone right there on the bus. Not many people had cell phones at that time and Randy looked very out of place making business arrangements. I had never before had someone move heaven and earth to be with me. I felt so special, so lucky for this sweet treatment.

Later that evening, we debated graduate school stipends, student loans for people pursuing degrees in professions that wouldn't afford the students a salary on which to pay back the loans, and so much more. We fit a lot in during that inexpensive Chinese dinner.

Randy was so handsome to me, but it takes more than looks to make one truly fall in love. I guess it must have been the combination of intellect and fun, geek and athlete, technology and the arts, honesty and integrity that drew me to him. I loved that he was a serious scientist and an intellectual, but not a snob. He didn't take himself too seriously, even though he voiced serious opinions and felt strongly about his convictions. He was full of life: that person who brings energy into the room and to whom you naturally gravitate. And the way he looked at me, even from the first moment, it was like nothing I had ever experienced before, and maybe never will again.

After that encounter, our romance was a whirlwind. He lived in Pittsburgh, Pennsylvania, and I in Chapel Hill, North Carolina, so naturally there was lots of travel involved to nurture the relationship. Sometimes I would travel up to Pittsburgh where he would show me the city, introduce me to friends and colleagues, and quietly begin to integrate me into his life. Love started to bloom, though I could not see it. I wasn't sure I could believe that such a man would be serious about me, about a woman who was already divorced at thirty and still working on her PhD in literature.

As our courtship continued into the fall, I brought him to my grandparents' home in Chesapeake, Virginia, for Thanksgiving. As a gift, he brought a gingerbread house for my grandmother that he'd made himself in the evenings after work. How surprising to find a man who baked and created gingerbread houses! And he did this from scratch and from a pattern he had made out of cardboard, not from a kit purchased at Michaels. The effort and attention he put into creating and transporting the house spoke volumes about him and the things he valued. He could have bought a bouquet of flowers to my family gathering, but Randy went the extra mile to make a good impression. It showed the real creative side of him, too, one that didn't *do* ordinary.

Later on, he took me to Columbia, Maryland, for his mother's and father's birthday celebrations. His gift to his father was simple: homemade chocolate chip cookies. In Randy's opinion, gifts weren't about showing how much money one was willing to spend, but rather about the amount of heart one put into it. His philosophy resonated with me, and I grew to love and respect him even more.

Soon we were spending every weekend and every holiday together, and Randy introduced me to some unforgettable experiences. It could be a behind-the-scenes tour of a theme park design at a popular amusement park or meeting people who were full of intriguing ideas. He invited me to come to business dinners and on business trips, even though I wasn't a computer scientist. I loved the intellectual stimulation, the conversations that challenged my preconceived notions, and the eclectic subject matter. Knowing I didn't have his technology background, Randy explained to me the basic ideas behind the subject at hand so I would be able to participate. He did this in a considerate, matter-of-fact way without any condescension. Moreover, he would ask me my opinion or impression, listening carefully, demonstrating how much he valued my input. As the weekends flew by, the weekdays stretched out longer and longer. It was getting harder not to be with the guy all the time. The distance between us couldn't be closed by a telephone call.

I vividly remember a field trip to Chicago with his Carnegie Mellon master's program students. We saw Blue Man Group for the first time together. One of the most unique theatrical performances today, Blue Man Group involves three actors painted blue from head to toe who never say a word on stage, but rather use drums, technology, and body language to communicate with and dazzle their audience. It was so novel, unlike any theatre we had ever experienced. At the end, Randy was blown away. He turned to me with tears in his eyes and said, "I'm so glad you were here to experience this with me." Later that night, we went to see *Tony and Tina's Wedding,* a play in which the audience is treated as guests at the wedding, even participating in the action. So when the actors called for all the single ladies to come up to catch the bouquet, Randy and his colleagues insisted I go up. To my surprise, I caught the bouquet. You can only imagine the ribbing we both got from his colleagues and students. After the trip to Chicago, I knew it wouldn't be long before Randy formally proposed to me. But I wasn't sure if I could let go of my fears and truly give my heart. I worried that I would be trapped once again in a marriage with a husband who would not work on problems but continue destructive behavior, and I would have to live unhappily or go through a painful divorce. Was I going to let my past cloud my future? Would I stay tied to that one failure or recognize my strength and try again? These were some of the questions I asked myself again and again.

He was fun, he was witty, but most important, he was caring. I knew he loved me because he showed me, not just told me. Randy's actions revealed his heart and character, in little ways, like buying me an umbrella when I didn't have one, or big ways, like promising me he would pay all expenses to move me back to Chapel Hill in the event our relationship soured. Though I had great trepidation, I trusted Randy and our relationship, and I agreed to move to Pittsburgh. I was still scared when I gave my two-week notice as outreach coordinator and office assistant at the Department of Computer Science, told my friends and family I was moving, and started looking for an apartment and job in Pittsburgh. Every time I drive up to Pittsburgh on I-70 W and the Pennsylvania Turnpike, I remember my trip with Randy in the U-Haul truck with all my worldly possessions packed in the back and car in tow. Those feelings of fear and excitement bubble up when I remember Randy behind the wheel, looking at me, smiling, reaching over to hold my hand. After one failed marriage, it took courage to trust someone again. But Randy made it easy for me to believe in him and in us. I knew our marriage would never end in divorce. I knew it was "until death do us part"; I just didn't know it would be so soon after uttering our vows. We were married on May 20, 2000, in Pittsburgh, under two large oak trees in a simple ceremony with just close family and a few friends in attendance.

Even after Dylan, Logan, and Chloe came along, the magic continued. Randy loved being a father and wanted enough children "to pile into the car," as he explained to me. I was thirty-four years old and Randy forty when we started our family. So there wasn't a lot of time between children. Dylan was born at the end of 2001. Logan came along two and a half years later, and Chloe nineteen months after Logan. Three children in five years! Small children put a lot of stress on a marriage, and ours was no exception. When Dylan was born seven weeks premature at two pounds fifteen ounces, Randy and I were terrified of losing our first child. I remember Randy went into his problem-solving mode to create a working schedule where my mom, me, and he all took turns getting up with Dylan every three hours to feed and change him, and record his input and output so the pediatrician could measure his growth, even going so far as to describe the consistency and color of his stool and how he ate. (I believe I still have some of these charts in a file. Imagine describing infant poop at three a.m.!) The danger when he was small was that he was too weak to cry when he needed food, so we did this for about three months straight until Dylan gained enough weight that we could wait for him to cry out when he was hungry. Very exhausting. I don't think Dylan ever slept through the night until he was about five years old and had learned to put on a story CD to listen to when he woke up in the middle of the night. We learned during this time that Randy did not do so well waking up in the middle of the night, for he couldn't get back to sleep and would then be exhausted in the morning before going to work. Because I could stay home and nap during the day when the children napped, I took over the night shifts to relieve Randy and make his life a little easier. Give and take. That's what we always did together to work through the tough times and to make our lives better together.

As I threw myself more deeply and completely into taking care of Dylan, Randy saw I was in danger of losing all boundaries between my tiny infant and me. Always self-assured, he believed he knew what I needed when I wasn't thinking straight because exhaustion and fear had colored my decision-making process. Seeing the rabbit hole I was down, he imposed time away from our baby and our house so that I would take a breath of air for myself. I did not like this arrangement at all but grudgingly left Dylan in his father's care. I remember going to a park and sitting there trying to read, unable to concentrate on the words on the page. All I could see was red—anger that I wasn't with Dylan. After a few more times, I learned

to extract myself from Mommy mode and use the couple of hours
to pursue some interests of my own. That newfound sense of self-
awareness and self-preservation served me well as our next two
children were born soon after and close together. It might not have
been what I wanted to hear or to see in myself, but Randy and I had
such open and honest communication that we could share anything
with each other. If one didn't agree with the other's point of view
or suggestion, we would respectfully disagree or find a compromise
that worked well enough for the both of us. I can remember only
a few times when we raised our voices in anger or frustration with
one another, which is remarkable, given the stress of child rearing
and a life-threatening illness. Randy was always so rational and reasonable, and he loved me so completely that he would do anything
for me.

Although the infant stage was hard for him, Randy really came
into his own when the children got to be about two years old. He
was the one who would do crazy things with them. One of their
favorite games was Scare the Mommy, which usually consisted of
silly tricks. When they were little, Randy liked to balance the kids
in the palm of his hand. The child would stand up straight as Randy
moved his hand up, down, and around. Of course, I would scream
and cry out at the appropriate moments, and the kids thought this
was great. Randy was also the one with whom they could curl up
on the couch. Mommy always seemed busy taking care of one child
or another or preparing some meal or snack, but Daddy was their
snuggle buddy, giving them lots of one-on-one attention, talking
with them about their day or some topic of interest. Randy also
cooked with them, mostly breakfast on the weekends, when we had
more leisure time. Randy's favorite thing to make was animal pancakes. He didn't use a preformed mold, but rather poured the mix

directly onto the skillet in such a way as to make a shape that kind of looked like something. It was the kids' job to determine what shape the pancake was, perhaps a horse or a pig. It was like a Rorschach test, a fun game that elicited much conversation and laughter at the breakfast table. We spent many a happy morning over those crazy pancakes!

As much as we loved spending time together, we also loved being with our families. We wanted the children to know both of our families, even though we lived at least four hours from our closest relative. So we would make trip after trip to Maryland and Virginia to visit, from the time the children were just babies. I remember the last family trip we took before Randy learned he had cancer. It was the summer of 2006, and we had decided to visit my younger brother in Raleigh, North Carolina. Most people would not see the combination of a newborn with a twenty-two-month-old and a four-and-a-half-year-old for a long road trip as their idea of a vacation. But we were committed to the idea of keeping our family ties close. Little did we know how much we would test those ties as we soon would call on our families to help us.

It was early August and the weather was hot—Southern hot, when the humidity hovers around 90 percent all the time and the day starts off at a cool 85 degrees. We stayed at a little hotel with a pool not far from my brother's house. The key word here is pool. During the few days we stayed in Raleigh, we spent most of the time in the water. The boys and Randy loved it; the two took turns jumping in, waiting for Randy to catch them, while I held baby Chloe in a more tranquil part of the pool. My brother and his wife came over to grill out in the evening and relax in the shade or play in the water with the kids. My friends from college came by to join us for a dip.

I particularly remember one friend watching Randy play with the boys; she was so touched by their love for each other and the joy they had being together. I remember looking at the same scene and thinking how happy I was that I was part of such a wonderful family and how many more times I would see this scene unfold in different ways throughout my lifetime: my husband, their father, loving them, being with them, enjoying the simple pleasures in life. This was one of my dreams come true: having a family—a loving, happy family. It had its challenges, no doubt, but the rewards were far greater than I ever expected. I loved being a mother and a wife, and I threw myself into these roles with fervor, learning how to grow my heart big enough to love four people. When life looks so rosy, it's hard to imagine the ground shaking and opening up to swallow you whole. The worst thing I could imagine at this time was one of the children having an ear infection. We couldn't know that our journey as a family and as a couple was about to take a serious turn—one that would test us and threaten to break us. What we had going for us was our strong bond and a love built on trust and communication. I think back on how I hesitated to leave my old life in Chapel Hill to build a new life with Randy in Pittsburgh. It was the right thing to do—to think carefully about marriage, knowing with 20/20 vision how difficult it is to maintain a healthy relationship. It's a decision I never regretted, even to this day.

2

Shattered Dreams

I<small>T WAS EARLY</small> in the morning on Labor Day weekend, September 2006, when we received a phone call from our general practitioner; he was following up on a CT scan that had been done of Randy's abdomen the previous day. The fact that the doctor would call us on a Saturday, much less a holiday weekend, didn't bode well. The feeling I had was the same as when the phone rings at midnight—a big knot in the pit of my stomach. "What does the doctor want to talk to me about?" I asked Randy as he held out the phone for me.

Though rarely sick, Randy had been feeling terrible for several weeks. We were trying to find the culprit for his mysterious symptoms: fatigue, weight loss, lack of appetite, floating stool. The obvious ailments, like flu, strep throat, hepatitis A, B, and C, had come back with negative test results.

With Randy unable to get out of bed, I had been pulling the night shift with the baby and the early-morning shift with the boys. Even having help with the kids during the week, I was getting run-down. Caring for the family, managing our house renovation project, and juggling several other commitments were beginning to take their toll. Like any couple, Randy and I had developed a routine, dividing the responsibilities and working with each other to keep the Pausch family train moving smoothly along its track.

Our typical day started early as Dylan, age four and a half, and Logan, twenty-three months, woke up around six o'clock each morning. Since I was nursing the baby and got up with four-month-old Chloe throughout the night, Randy would get up with the boys and make breakfast. Dylan would often stand on a step stool and help Randy cook, enjoying the thrill of helping out in the kitchen by breaking or scrambling eggs. Logan would play contently with toys until it was time to eat. After I came downstairs with Chloe, we would have breakfast together. Then Randy would get ready for work and start his day at the university.

My primary responsibilities included the children and our house renovations. We were raising the roof on our ranch house in Pittsburgh to give us a little extra room as our family grew. At this time, I was picking out fixtures, from plumbing items to tile, as well as tweaking the design. We were working with a great building contractor and architect who did all the heavy lifting and were very trustworthy, but I still needed to decide on the details, like the location of light switches and the number and location of outlets in a room. I also oversaw a wonderful nanny, Amy Samad, who helped me with the children and their activities. Amy gave me the opportunity to sit down every once in a while and not run myself ragged. With doctor visits, preschool, child-centered activities like music classes, and household management, there was more than enough work to go around. Just keeping up with laundry and meals for three little ones under the age of five took up hours every day.

While I assumed the domestic responsibilities, Randy managed the family finances, taking care of bills and taxes. He also liked to suggest and arrange our travel, usually getting us to go with him on trips where the family would enjoy the location. Whenever he consulted with Walt Disney Company, Inc., we would try to go along. My part of the travel arrangements involved packing the necessary clothes, snacks, and toys for the trip. In addition, Randy focused on his career, which included teaching classes, advising PhD and master's students throughout their academic careers, leading his research team, writing grant applications, attending and presenting at conferences, collaborating with other researchers, attending various academic department meetings, and participating in hiring decisions. He wore many different hats and enjoyed the diverse demands of the job. I don't think people realize all the components of a professor's job, but there's much more to it besides teaching and conducting research. Randy loved his job, especially at Carnegie Mellon University, to the point that he felt indebted to the institution for all the opportunities it had given him.

On the home front, Randy and I had developed a symbiotic relationship in which each of us contributed to our family life and to raising our children. Both our parts were crucial to making it work. I valued Randy tremendously for his efforts and I know he valued me for mine. He was a large cog in the wheel; without him, the delicate balance of maintaining our family was thrown out of whack. The train was off its track and bumping noisily and dangerously along. Our family sorely felt his absence when he had to travel for business, which was about a week each month, or put in the long hours necessary for his job. Randy used to joke about the job flexibility offered by the university, saying he could work his eighty hours a week any time he wanted.

The present moment would help crystallize just how much we all leaned on Randy. As he held out his cell phone for me, I was mystified why the doctor would want to talk to me. "He wants to tell you himself," Randy said as I sat down on the floor with phone in hand. What the doctor had to tell me was that there was a mass on Randy's pancreas that was most likely cancer. I remember the doctor telling me it wasn't fair and how sorry he was, but I don't remember what else he said. I didn't bother to ask him what the pancreas did or where it was located. I didn't ask about survival rates. I was just too stunned, too shocked by the word *cancer*. Randy was just shy of his forty-sixth birthday! I can't even remember the end of the conversation. What I do remember so clearly was watching Randy during the phone call and studying his expression, looking for clues from the man I admired most as to what the hell was happening. I knew this was bad news, I just couldn't figure out how bad.

After hanging up, I came over to the bed and handed Randy his cell phone. I kept my eyes on his face the entire time. His handsome, boyish face was so serious, his brown eyes intensely focused. I could only guess at the calculations going on in that wonderful, intelligent brain of his. Then, with a steady, authoritative voice, the man of my dreams told me matter-of-factly he was going to die. Moreover, he probably had only three to six months to live. All this he had learned from googling "pancreatic cancer" on his laptop in bed. There wasn't an ounce of self-pity in his voice, just a quiet acknowledgment of the facts as he understood them now. As if intuiting how critical time was for him, Randy went to work to find a loophole in death's contract, not so much for himself, but for me and for his children. If there was a ray of hope out there, Randy was determined to find it and grab hold.

Looking back on this scene now, I can see how this situation would become the new norm for Randy: sitting in bed working on his laptop and/or talking on his cell phone. Instead of going to his university office or into the classroom as the dynamic teacher and researcher he was, he would conduct all his work from our bed. His laptop, once my rival for his attention, would become his lifeline, keeping him connected to his research group, his students, colleagues, family, and doctors. In this way, Randy was able to continue doing so many of the things he loved even as cancer slowly took away his energy.

Except for the yellow tinge to his skin caused by the tumor pressing against his bile duct and causing bilirubin to build up in his bloodstream, Randy looked perfectly healthy. How could he know for sure he was going to die? How could he be so sure? I was reeling from the verbal blows. The jabs from the doctor and Randy left me dizzy, my head spinning. I was trying to process all this new information, trying to hold on to the marvelous life we had built together in eight short years, which was now suddenly so fragile.

Since we met in the fall of 1998, Randy and I had put down roots together in Pittsburgh because of his job. We developed a network of close friends with whom we got together for dinner, movies, concerts, sporting events, and plays. We celebrated children's birthdays and holidays together. We had found a church where we both felt comfortable and went every Sunday we were in town. We were involved in each other's professional lives. When I was working, Randy would look over my web designs, make suggestions, and show me user testing techniques. On the flip side, I helped host parties at our house for his students and attended university functions with him. We played flag football together in the Pittsburgh Sports League as Randy taught me the rules of the game and how to rush the quarterback. I played even after Dylan was born, nursing him on the sidelines during halftime, but quit a short time later. Randy continued to play for several years and we maintained friendships with our teammates.

The most significant thing we had done was start a family together. My first pregnancy had been difficult. At a seven-month checkup, the doctor became concerned by how infrequently I felt the baby move. I was sent to the hospital for an ultrasound which showed that Dylan was very small for his gestational age and that his legs were up around his ears in the frank breech birth position, which contributed to his lack of movement. The biggest issue was his weight. Our obstetrician recommended bed rest, daily fetal monitoring, and a series of steroid shots to help accelerate his lung development. The concern was that Dylan would come early and be unable to breathe, because a baby's lungs are the last organs to develop. Randy was very calm during these meetings, always holding my hand and providing me with the emotional support I needed during this time. He did become a little rattled when my placenta partially detached and bright red blood soaked my underpants. Not only did he break the speed limit and run red lights to get me to the hospital, but he almost ran over my mother when she didn't get out of the car fast enough. Randy held my hand throughout the emergency Cesarean surgery. When I hovered on the brink of shock, he kept me from going over the edge. He stayed beside me in the recovery room as the medication wore off and the pain kicked in letting me know how unhappy my body was with the trauma it had just experienced. The two of us celebrated the arrival of 2002 thankful to have a premature baby weighing only two pounds fifteen ounces lying in the neonatal intensive care unit some floors below us. Dylan's wasn't the last difficult pregnancy and birth we would endure together, but it was the first medical crisis that would test our mettle and teach us to rely utterly and completely on each other.

When I needed to see Dylan in the neonatal intensive care unit, Randy would drive me there regardless of the time of day or night. He loved that little guy just as much as I did and we shared kangaroo duty, placing Dylan against our bare skin to help him to thrive. And thrive he did, gaining weight and normalizing his heartbeat and breathing. After twenty-one days in neonatal intensive care, our baby weighed three and a half pounds and was ready to come home. The neonatal team encouraged us to spend the night in a special bedroom with Dylan off the monitors so Randy and I would feel confident when we walked out those hospital doors and took our child home. Randy, I, and the staff had become dependent on the heart monitor to tell us Dylan was OK. When they removed the pads from Dylan's tiny chest, we both held our breath hoping that he wouldn't suddenly go into distress. As the minutes went by, we slowly began to breathe normally. Before the hospital staff left us alone for the evening, they pointed out the emergency cord we could pull if we felt Dylan needed medical attention. A nurse would come to our rescue if we needed her. That emergency cord made us feel a little more comfortable, but we were very nervous that first night in the hospital room.

We made it through the early days and months of having a premature baby who needed to be awakened every three hours for feedings. Adding a baby to our relationship came with its own set of challenges as we balanced being parents with keeping our love and marriage strong. We struggled as a couple during the first couple of years, as I threw myself into being a mother and didn't give Randy the time and attention he needed. There were many heart-to-heart discussions and some tears. The great thing about our marriage was that we could have these soul-baring talks without either of us letting our emotions get the better of us and saying hurtful things that we would regret later. We never raised our voices in anger at each other. We were both committed to making our marriage work and I knew beyond a shadow of a doubt that he wouldn't walk away or give up on us.

When I found out I was pregnant with Logan we were living in San Mateo, California, where Randy was doing a sabbatical with Electronic Arts, a company that makes video games. A sabbatical is a special academic privilege that a professor may be awarded once every seven years or so, going off from his or her classes and university duties to do something intellectually enriching. Randy's first sabbatical had been with Walt Disney Imagineering. Now he was working with the video gaming giant to get a better understanding of the gaming industry's culture. Halfway through my pregnancy the sabbatical ended and we moved east to our home in Pittsburgh. During one of my prenatal checkups, my urine test showed alarmingly high levels of protein. The doctor told me to go right to the hospital; they needed to do more tests because I was showing signs of preeclampsia, and they might need to induce labor. I was so frightened, so scared that we were going to have a repeat emergency delivery and something would be wrong with the baby. To make matters worse, I had two-year-old Dylan with me and I couldn't register at the hospital with him in tow.

I called Randy, who was in a really important meeting, to explain the dilemma we were in. My husband didn't hesitate and left the meeting immediately to be by my side. He called a sitter to take care of Dylan while he stayed with me at the hospital. Together we

waited while the doctors performed one test after another, not giving us any indication which way the situation was going: were my
liver and kidneys beginning to fail, forcing them to induce labor?
Many hours later, the doctors told us I was going to be OK, and we
could breathe a sigh of relief.

Logan did come a couple of week's early, and I was diagnosed
with preeclampsia when I went into labor on October 2, 2004. My
labor stalled as a result of the medicine the doctor gave me to keep
me from having a seizure. The doctor gave us the option of electing
to deliver via C-section or trying for a natural birth. Randy and I
talked for a few minutes and when the doctor returned we said we
wanted to go natural. Big mistake! After pushing for an hour Logan
got stuck in the birth canal. Off to the OR we went with medical
personnel flooding the room. Our intimate birthing experience was
suddenly swapped out for the drama of an assisted birthing procedure. Logan was too far down the birth canal for a C-section, so the
doctor and his assistant used forceps to pull while two nurses on either side of my belly pushed down as hard as they could as I pushed
during a contraction. When Logan's head emerged, we thought his
body would just slip out, but that didn't happen and the doctor had
to gently pull some more until the baby came free. I remember
allowing myself to drift away and lose consciousness after hearing
Logan's healthy cries. I knew the doctors and nurses would take
care of him. When I opened my eyes a few moments later, they were
still hovering around the baby and I noticed that no one would let
me see him. I asked Randy to let me see the baby, but he wouldn't
do it, saying I could see him later. Instinctively I knew something
was wrong and I demanded Randy tell me what was going on. He
said Logan's shoulder had been damaged during the birth. Perhaps a
nerve had been pinched. Whatever it was, Logan wasn't moving his

arm or shoulder and we didn't know whether the damage was temporary or permanent. As I lay there on the table while the doctor stitched me up, terror squeezed my heart as my conscience tortured me: Oh God, how I regretted my decision to go through a natural birth instead of the C-section! I accused myself of being selfish and putting my child at risk. After a while, Randy happily told me Logan was beginning to move his shoulder and that he would be all right. Throughout the ordeal, Randy had stood by my side, never offering a word of criticism or casting doubt or blame. He was simply there for me and I knew I could lean on him.

As our family grew, the demands placed on Randy's time became more problematic. Traveling a week out of each month was exacting a greater cost on our family. Like most couples, Randy and I discussed how to balance work versus family. At times I felt I was raising our children alone as he was either traveling or working in the lab, at the university or in our home office. His thoughts were often consumed by work—or at least that's how I felt. Randy wanted to cut back on some of his academic responsibilities, but the question was where. He had several graduate students he was advising on their PhDs, which took up a lot of time one-on-one with them. He had to meet the requirements laid out in his grant contracts until the award period was over. He could reduce the number of talks he gave, but he wasn't willing to give that up completely, because he enjoyed putting together his talks, as well as delivering them. Finally he landed on his commitment to various academic departments. After much thought and discussion, Randy decided to give up the codirectorship of the Entertainment Technology Center, an academic center he had helped found. It brought together students from various disciplines to collaborate and offered a master's degree in entertainment technology. Shortly after Randy cut back his schedule, his father was diagnosed with a rare form of leukemia for which there is no cure. Randy was able to use his extra time to spend with his father as well as his still growing family as I was pregnant with our third child. Increasing family demands forced Randy and me to have some heart-to-heart discussions about our life priorities. I wanted him to be able to focus on us when he was with us and not have his mind swirling around problems at work. I also wanted him to be with us more often and travel less. As the children grew older and started to play sports, I wanted Randy to coach them, giving them the positive experience he had as a child when he played little-league football.

Randy wanted these things too, but it was honestly difficult for him to turn down the intellectually interesting opportunities that came up at work. I understood his dilemma, having had to make the decision to give up my career the year after Dylan was born. I had worked and earned my own money since seventh grade, working on a neighborhood farm or doing yard work, then minimum-wage jobs after I turned sixteen. Knowing I was totally dependent on Randy for our financial well-being was a leap of faith on my part. I didn't realize at the time how much I gave up in terms of intellectual challenge, but I was able to find ways to keep my brain stimulated. Through his job, Randy enjoyed creativity and teaching. I understood that once he gave up being a director of an academic center or an instructor of a popular college course, he would in all likelihood not be able to reverse his decisions later. So we did not make any rash decisions that we might regret later on and kept talking together to find the balance that worked for our family.

In light of where we were in our lives—late thirties/early forties, raising three small children—a life-threatening illness was nowhere on our radar. I quickly learned there's no scarier pronouncement

than "You have cancer," unless it's "Your loved one has cancer." I had
previously known only one other person with cancer: an acquain-
tance from church. No one in either of our families had had cancer
that required chemo or radiation. So I didn't have a frame of refer-
ence to help guide me in this moment or down the road on our
cancer odyssey. Because that's where we were: on a new road in life,
one that would challenge us individually and test the strength of our
love and our commitment to each other.

Looking at Randy, listening to his prediction, processing the doctor's words, I didn't realize I was watching my dream shatter in
real time. I wanted to cling to the beauty and security of our normal life, but that life was like a broken stained-glass window, lying
about my feet in shards. In my ignorance I thought if we could just
get through this cancer thing, if Randy could just beat the odds,
our lives would go back to normal. I didn't understand that even if
Randy did beat the cancer, our lives would never go back to what
they were because cancer would always be lurking in the shadows,
hiding around the corner. Instead, there was a new normal now and
its name was fear.

Night after night I would lie in bed on the third floor listening
to the baby making her little noises and thinking about what was
happening. After I knew the baby had nursed and would sleep for
a bit, I would slip down to the second floor and find Randy equally
awake. We would hold each other, and I would cry. Randy would
reassure me that I could raise the children on my own, that I could
manage the finances. He didn't cry for himself, but rather for us, for
the family he had created and knew he wouldn't be around to help
raise. He cried for me and for the arduous task ahead of me. What a
sad sight the sun rose to each of those mornings!

I don't know how I functioned those days with so little sleep, nursing a baby every three hours, trying to make life seem normal for the boys, planning with the builder to finish our renovations as quickly as possible, meeting with doctors to discuss Randy's treatment and provide him with the best chance at survival. I guess that's the biggest lesson I had to learn—and relearn—throughout this journey: to trust myself to face the challenges set before me. One has to dig down deep, but there it is waiting to be released: an untapped well of can-do. I've seen people I've known rise to face all sorts of obstacles I would never think myself capable of overcoming. So when I found myself in similar circumstances, I realized I just had to do what needed to be done. What were my options, really? Turn my back on Randy, the man who had loved me, cared for me, and helped create a life of happiness and completeness?

I recently heard a wonderful sermon at my church during which our ministers talked about marriage vows; how we have to find the meaning behind the vow and strive to fulfill it every day. Minister John Manwell said, "It takes only a few moments to make the vow, but a lifetime to live it." Randy used to say something more playful, "Marry in haste; repent at leisure." I did not regret marrying Randy even in the face of his death. I believe he felt the same about me, even though I occasionally failed him throughout his ordeal. Still, we loved each other and I tried my best to fulfill my vows.

3

Face the Problem

JUST AS I REACTED with shock and disbelief to the news of Randy's cancer, so did our family members. To help them process all that the diagnosis entailed, Randy sent an e-mail reiterating the pertinent information. As always, Randy was calm and methodical as he addressed the immediate impact and ongoing threat cancer created in our lives. He did not resort to fear mongering to heighten the drama or to drum up support from his family. Instead, he maintained a positive outlook and chose to focus on the possibilities, however slim. Here's what he wrote on September 12, 2006:

> Jai & I are overwhelmed by the rapid and heartfelt offers of help, which we fully intend to say "yes" to! (see next message).
>
> First, in this message, I'd like to give you all a little information about the disease, and put a few potential fears

at rest. I hate using email, but it has the nice feature that everyone hears me say exactly the same thing.

1) Although the diagnosis is scary, I am NOT planning on dying anytime soon! You all need to know that Jai & I are committed to beating the odds, strengthened by our love for each other and the loving support of our families.

2) I want to make very clear that if I should die, Jai and the children will NOT be a financial burden on any of you. We have savings, a paid-for house, and I have life insurance with Carnegie Mellon and external companies that will financially protect Jai if I die. She will need your emotional support, but not your financial support. I met with Carnegie Mellon's president yesterday, and they will be keeping me on full salary throughout this entire process, and helping in any way they can.

3) I thought I would share specific information about the disease I have: My diagnosis is adenocarcinoma, a cancer of the pancreas. Usually this cancer is found so late that they send people home to die within 3–6 months.

Fortunately, I'm one of the 20% of patients where the surgeons can remove the tumor. I'm scheduled for surgery on Tuesday, Sept 19th at UPMC Shadyside Hospital. It's a major surgery, where they will remove my tumor, my gallbladder, part of my pancreas, part of my small intestine, and possibly part of my stomach. I will be in the hospital 2–3 weeks, and then another 4 weeks of bed rest at home. At that point, I'll be physically 100% again.

We have done extensive research, and Jai & I are very happy with my surgeon (who has done over 250 of these operations), and the facility here, which is considered

a "high volume" center for this procedure. The surgery,
by the way, is called a "Whipple" procedure, after its
inventor.

If the surgery removes every last cancer cell, I win.
Otherwise, eventually the cancer will come back. Statistically, the long-term prognosis is not rosy; only 10–20% of
people who have the surgery survive to five years. Needless to say, I intend to be one of the lucky ones who sticks
around! The median age for this disease is 66 and so there
is some reason to believe my odds will be better than the
typical patient's (I'm 45 and in good physical shape), so
they can hit me with more aggressive chemotherapy and/
or radiation after the surgery.

Jai & I are now completely focused on the short term,
and taking care of the kids.

I love Randy's message; it makes me smile every time I read it
because it exemplifies his spirit and positive outlook in a dire situation. In his e-mail, the first thing Randy did was to accept and
acknowledge the facts. He didn't shy away from the "C" word or the
stark reality of the disease. There isn't an ounce of self-pity or a hint
of depression. He doesn't come across as angry or morose because
he never was—not once. More important, Randy doesn't sound
like a man who is giving up, but rather like a general organizing his
battle plan and alerting the troops. His message was reassuring to
his extended family and in-laws, but it's not a glossed-over version
of the truth. He doesn't distort the facts to make up some fairy-tale
version of what we were facing. I vividly remember him saying he
wanted to send this e-mail to everyone in our family at the same
time so that there wouldn't be a version of the telephone game

as one family member called another and gave inaccurate information. What they did with that information afterward was beyond his control, but at least he had given them clear and truthful data on his part.

He was also clear on the delicate topic of finances. We didn't talk about money with our families, but this situation warranted broaching the subject. By nature, Randy was a frugal person. Even as a graduate student living on a meager stipend he had managed to save money. By the time we had met, he had built up a nice nest egg. As we combined our lives and our incomes, we made sure to add to our savings and retirement accounts, never living outside of our means. Now our prudence would pay off big time. Knowing his family was provided for in the worst-case scenario took a huge weight off Randy's shoulders, allowing him to focus on his health and treatment. I think it also was a source of pride as the result of his hard work and planning. I, too, was also able to breathe a huge sigh of relief, because the salary I made before I stopped working would never cover the bills and pay for day care and after-school care. Although we were humble in asking our families to help us through Randy's surgical recovery and treatments, at least we didn't have to walk up to their door hat in hand, asking for money.

There are many ways people respond to bad news, and especially to a life-threatening illness. Some give in to their emotions for a period of time. I know I reacted emotionally to hearing that Randy had an aggressive form of cancer that had an 80 percent chance of killing him the first year. Behind closed doors, away from family and friends, Randy and I would support each other as we vented our feelings and fears. We didn't keep them bottled up, but rather found safe ways to express them. I found that talking to close friends about my feelings or some upsetting change in our predicament helped me tremendously. We were never paralyzed by our emotions to the point that we couldn't function or address the situation.

It is important to note that some cancers do not afford you the luxury of sitting idly by for days, weeks, or months. We quickly realized that we were now on cancer time, in which each minute of every hour counted as never before. Regardless of how slim the chance, we grabbed for the brass ring before the window of opportunity closed. By acting quickly, by doing our homework, and by educating ourselves about the most effective treatments, we were helping to shape our journey. If we had remained paralyzed with fear or chosen not to act, we could have lost traction in the fight against the cancer and lost precious time for Randy to live.

At this point, the cancer wasn't exacting a terrible toll on Randy's body. He had jaundice, and the buildup of bilirubin in his blood made him itchy all over. Since I had bitten my nails to the nubs, my mom scratched his back until there were red marks all over it. All the while, Randy sighed at having some relief from the itching. I think learning what had been causing his lethargy and other symptoms actually made him feel a little better. Randy was a doer. Just the fact that he could do something now—like research the disease and treatments—perked him up. Though his energy level wasn't what it had been, he still functioned normally for the most part. He wasn't eating as much and had stopped exercising all together. But he met with people throughout the day and worked on his computer on various projects. He made sure his PhD student was in a good place and that his life insurance had the correct wording on the beneficiary in case he died either during the surgery or due to complications afterward.

Part of improving Randy's odds for survival involved finding a surgeon who was experienced in performing the difficult proce-

dure. The surgeon needed to be affiliated with a hospital with a recovery center well versed in helping the patient recover and dealing
with the various complications that typically arise after the surgery.
All these factors were important to consider because the mortality
rate from the surgery alone can be as high as 20 percent or as low
as 5 percent. Reducing Randy's risk in as many ways as possible was
at the forefront of our minds. We were fortunate in having an excellent surgeon, Dr. Herbert Zeh, and Shadyside hospital was well
equipped to help Randy recuperate right in Pittsburgh. With the
next step in battle against the cancer decided, we then turned our
attention to me to address the real possibility of physical and emotional exhaustion.

In his second e-mail, also sent on September 12, 2006, Randy
elaborated on the dangers of overloading me as the family's primary
caregiver:

> Our biggest concern is making sure that Jai has help. For
> two months starting Sept 19th, she will not only be do-
> ing the job of a single parent with a 4-year-old (Dylan),
> 23-month-old (Logan), and nursing four-month-old
> (Chloe), she will be doing so while either visiting me in
> the hospital or while I'm recovering at home.
>
> Jai is one of the strongest women I've ever met, but
> she's human, and the task before her is Herculean. We
> must avoid Jai "burn-out" at all costs.
>
> Our basic plan is to use local help Monday–Friday (we
> think we have a good plan in place), and to accept all of
> your offers of help to come visit for weekends. It would
> be most helpful if people could come here, arriving by

Friday afternoon/evening, and leaving Monday. We will
have plenty of room to put up visitors.

Jai will be talking with you in the next 48 hours to set
up a calendar to make sure we have full coverage; my family will be doing what they can, as well.

God bless you all for your willingness to help in what is
truly our time of need.

In addition to educating ourselves about pancreatic cancer and
treatment options, I think one of the smartest things we did was to
acknowledge the impact cancer would have on our family. So often
people focus only on the patient, but cancer takes its toll on more
than that one person. As Randy so gallantly said at one point, I was
one tough broad, but I am only human. We knew that the stress,
combined with the situation's demands, created a strong probability
of wearing me down. So we planned on a support system for me so
I could best take care of my husband and our children, in hopes also
of keeping our marriage intact. Unfortunately, many oncologists
and cancer centers do not offer support for the patient's caregiver.
And caregivers can quickly find themselves overwhelmed without
the resources to help. I had never been in this position before, not
for a family member or friend. Taking my lack of experience into
consideration, we made sure to get ahead of the problem and ask
family and friends to come help us with patient care, child care,
meals, and domestic responsibilities, such as laundry.

With our family informed and a game plan in place, we now
focused on how and what to tell our children. At four months old,
obviously Chloe was too young to understand anything that was
going on. Trying to explain cancer to a two-year-old was not go-

ing to be an in-depth conversation, so we kept it short and sweet; Logan could understand very simply that Randy had a boo-boo and needed to see the doctor. That was all he could process and all he needed. Dylan was a different story. Though only four and a half years old, Dylan was not only perceptive, but he was able to understand complex topics. Here was a child who would devour information about dinosaurs, from how they lived, how large they were and what they ate, to how they died and what animals evolved from them. He would sit and listen quietly to the informational videos at the natural history museum while scientists in the film discussed the connection between birds and dinosaurs or the theories about the demise of the dinosaurs at the end of the Cretaceous Period. Given his precocious intelligence, it wouldn't be enough to tell Dylan that Daddy had a boo-boo. When we were ready, we took Dylan to a quiet room where we wouldn't be interrupted by his siblings, and we told him his father had a disease called cancer. We explained that he couldn't catch cancer like a cold. Randy explained that cancer was like a weed that grows in the garden. The weed grows and multiplies in the garden choking off the other plants and keeping them from getting the nutrients of the soil. Even though we pull the weeds out of the garden, they sometimes grow back after a period of time. Like the weeds, cancer was growing in Daddy's body and the doctor had to pull it out so it didn't continue to make Daddy feel sick. Dylan quickly asked Randy if he was going to die and Randy assured him he would not. After lots of hugs for reassurance, followed by a few more questions, Dylan hopped down off the bed and went to play with his brother. Randy and I sat there emotionally drained from the experience, leaning on each other for support until we could stand up once again and face the next set of challenges.

Randy's willingness to discuss his disease and treatments in a realistic yet hopeful manner throughout his battle with cancer was a huge upside for me and our family. As an engineer, Randy tended to focus on numbers and percentages, but he was also able to engage on an emotional level and discuss his feelings most of the time. Not everyone affected by cancer is as open as Randy. Some people don't want to know anything about the disease's progress or to weigh the options of the various treatments. A patient's denial can put a relative and/or caregiver in a terrible position, knowing what is going on but not being able to talk about the situation, about the feelings and fears a terminal illness conjures up, or about how to deal with impending death. In one case, my friend's husband chose to remain ignorant of the cancer's progress. The doctors respected his wish not to know about the disease and, as a result, met clandestinely with his wife, warning her how much longer her husband had to live. Then she suffered alone. Imagine her dilemma: she hears terrible news from the doctor in the hallway outside the examining room but has to go back to her loved one and put on a front of ignorant bliss. I feel so fortunate that Randy wanted to know and to have a hand in making decisions about his medical treatment, his hospice care, and even his funeral. Because he was so open with me I was able to understand the reasoning behind his choices and voice my agreement or trepidation. We didn't hide anything from each other. Maybe we didn't always like hearing what the other person said, but we always knew we were a team. We would support each other and that comforted us in a time of so much uncertainty and pain.

Randy's greatest strengths were his analytical skills and his ability to focus on solving a problem. However, sometimes too much of a good thing can turn into a negative. For Randy, the news that he had cancer threw him into engineering mode: assess situation, learn options, analyze data, and make informed decision with highest probability to solve problem. Intellectually Randy knew he had a very strong chance of dying and he did not shy away from the ugly statistics. His concern for my well-being and our family's future greatly weighed on his mind. If he couldn't beat the cancer, he would position his family as best he could for a future without him. Having identified the objective, Randy went to work analyzing the situation, putting full power to his brain and setting aside his feelings. The upside to his strategy was, he didn't become morose or hysterical. The downside was, his pragmatism could appear cold and uncaring. Sometimes he could say things to me that cut deeply into my heart, as when he questioned my decision-making abilities because I was a humanities major in college and not a trained scientist. As his health became more compromised, Randy relied heavily on his intellect and the army of knowledgeable people who helped us. He trusted his trained mind and felt the way he approached a problem was the best way to tackle it. Sometimes that caused friction between us.

Randy gave way to a certain imperiousness when I took over the checkbook and bill paying. The family finances had always been his responsibility. With his surgery date fast approaching, he felt it imperative that I learn all about our checking, savings, retirement accounts, taxes, online access passwords, and household budget formulas. Randy kept all our checking account information in an Excel spreadsheet, which he had designed himself, discarding the bank's paper check registry. He was very knowledgeable with Excel; I was not. His checking document was extremely complex, far beyond my abilities, but Randy insisted that I master his way of balancing the checkbook. His overbearing demeanor was out of character, but I think the fear he felt brought out the taskmaster in him. Was it really necessary that I learn Randy's Excel spreadsheet? No. I would have to develop my own system for managing our finances in a way that worked for me. But my learning his system gave Randy great peace of mind, relieving some of the tension he felt. Stress and uncertainty can bring about extreme behaviors and attitudes in a person and make things difficult for his or her loved ones. At the time, Randy and I were unskilled in recognizing when fear was driving our actions and how to cope with the stress.

Randy's anxieties over getting his affairs in order before the surgery were fueled by the possibility of dying either during or recovering from the procedure. Even though he had a greater chance of living than dying and even though we had found an excellent, experienced surgeon and recovery center, Randy wanted to do as much as possible for his family to ease our burden just in case the worst possible scenario came to pass. One of Randy's favorite sayings was, "Plan for the worst; hope for the best." One aspect that greatly concerned him was single parenthood for me: raising three small children in a city without any family nearby. I believe he felt very guilty about my difficult situation, even though it wasn't his fault. Moreover, he believed that children needed two parents to raise them, that they would be better cared for because there would be two sets of hands—and more patience.

Early in September 2006, Randy approached me about a possible solution to relieve some pressure from me and improve our children's quality of life. I remember him coming into the room, head down, avoiding my eyes—very unlike Randy. He prefaced the conversation by saying he knew I would say no, but he wanted me to hear him out. And then he asked me to think about giving up our daughter, our four-month-old baby, for adoption, as a way to ease my burden and give the children a better chance of having a better childhood with more attention and more love. His words struck me like a punch in the gut. It sickened me to even think of losing Chloe and I vehemently said no. He instantly acquiesced, never challenging my choice, and never brought it up again.

Now if you had ever told me before this moment that Randy would one day suggest giving up one of his children, I would have told you you were crazy!—that Randy would *never* do that. But Randy was focused on solving a problem, shelving his emotions so as not to color his vision. I think Randy could see how his death would leave his children at a disadvantage and I believe he was trying to find a way to deal them a better hand than the one they held. Maybe he could see the inevitable struggles I would have in functioning as a single parent; even before the cancer he and I both were already finding it difficult to care for three young children. His "solution" had nothing to do with how he felt about his daughter, for I know deep in my heart that Randy loved Chloe and under normal circumstances would never have contemplated giving her or any of our children up for adoption. He had wanted to have a third child after Logan was born, and he was delighted we had a healthy baby girl. He loved his daughter and his sons equally, loved being a father to them. But cancer introduced a level of stress so severe that Randy and I both struggled to cope. For his part, his singular drive to make us safe pushed him to extreme behavior and judgment. I knew he didn't want to lose Chloe any more than he wanted to die. Cancer and its power to kill him were the catalysts for his extreme request.

Learning how to manage the overwhelming feelings and stress one experiences while dealing with cancer takes awareness and coping skills, neither of which we developed until further along our cancer odyssey. The relationship between husband and wife, parent and child, becomes strained, pushed sometimes to the breaking point. As the caregiver, I felt like I was asked to make concessions and sacrifices for my husband and my children. It was a delicate balance to not lose all of myself in the swirl of fear and waves of strong emotions.

At the beginning of our journey, in addition to my usual role as mother and wife, I was adding another: emotional backstop and sounding board for a sick and potentially dying man. I had no idea what brick walls lay before me, but I knew I'd face any challenge to help my husband and care for my children. It was the least I could do for Randy, who had given me so much happiness and helped me become a better person. I admired and respected him, and I would not shy away from the new demands set before me to help him, regardless of the cost. How little did I know at that time how high the cost would be—or how great the rewards.

4

Shuttling Between My Husband and My Children

I'M SURE WE LOOKED LIKE a romantic couple to the neighbors as we walked along the sidewalk of our Pittsburgh neighborhood holding hands in the fall of 2006, leaning on each other, speaking softly. Instead of saying sweet nothings, we were strategizing how to maximize Randy's chances to beat pancreatic cancer and live to see his children grow up. For the couple of weeks following the discovery of the tumor, the September weather was nice and mild. Pittsburgh is such a beautiful place to be in the fall as the summer heat abates and the cool evenings set in. The turning leaves put on a spectacular show not just in the mountains, but in the city neighborhoods as well. During these solitary walks together, we didn't notice the trees or enjoy the change of seasons, but rather discussed various cancer regimens, where the providers were located, and the implications for our family in choosing treatment at a center far from home. I wish we had known about the Pancreatic Cancer Action Network, which through its Patients and Liaison Service provides support to newly diagnosed patients by connecting them with a trained associate who has information about oncologists and surgeons in the patient's area, up-to-date treatment options for pancreatic cancer, and even clinical trials conducted around the country. We would have saved so much time and energy by tapping into that wealth of information. Instead, Randy and his Carnegie Mellon colleague and friend, Jessica Hodgins, scoured the Internet for information on what options existed. They compared survival rates, the number of study participants, and blogs where patients and caregivers post about their experiences with doctors and drugs. Between the two of them, no stone was left unturned.

Randy began his treatment plan with the Whipple procedure, which was his Golden Ticket. Just by making it into the category of people eligible for surgery, Randy increased his odds of survival. In Randy's mind, that slim chance could then be converted into a touchdown for the team. The morning of September 19, 2006, I quietly nursed the baby at around four a.m. After I returned her to her crib, I dressed and left with Randy for the hospital, located just a few blocks away from our house. My mother and, later on, Amy stayed with the children. We arrived around five thirty a.m. I remember the hospital lights glaringly bright in contrast to the darkness of early dawn. We were taken upstairs where Randy was prepped for surgery. His clothes and other belongings were handed to me in a white plastic bag. I stayed by his bedside surrounded by a privacy curtain, holding his hand and whispering words of love and encouragement. We kissed briefly after the anesthesiologist came in to wheel him away with a quick promise to take good care of Randy. I allowed myself only a few minutes to cry alone before heading downstairs to the waiting area. Our family and friends would be coming soon, and I'd need to be there to keep them informed.

Randy's surgery lasted eight hours—a good sign that the cancer hadn't spread. The surgeon had told me beforehand that if, after opening Randy up, they saw that the cancer had spread beyond the pancreas, they would close him up and send him home to get his affairs in order. Happily, that was not the case. After removing the tumor, part of the pancreas, part of the stomach, some of the small intestines, a section of the small intestine called the duodenum, the gallbladder, part of the middle of the small intestine called the jejunum, the bile duct, and the lymph nodes near the pancreas, the surgeon sewed Randy up and sent him off to the intensive care unit to begin his difficult recovery.

As soon as Randy was home after a two-week recovery in the hospital, we moved to the second line of attack. Like other cancers, pancreatic cancer is usually treated with chemotherapy and/or radiation. Our local cancer center offered the standard of care, which meant treating Randy with a chemotherapy drug called gemcitabine. Unfortunately, this treatment meant a low probability of being alive in twelve months! Randy knew there were experimental treatments offered at cancer centers far from our home, but he was leaning toward staying in Pittsburgh for our family's convenience. Then one of his good friends took him aside and counseled him to reconsider his line of thinking; he explained that Randy was doing himself a disservice by not going to where the best treatment was. When you are trying to beat a tough opponent like a cancer that gives no second chances, your best strategy is to go to a facility with the treatment that offers the greatest chances of survival. You don't have the luxury of choosing where that treatment is located; rather, you focus on the results of the latest medical research. Pancreatic cancer is highly aggressive and resists most of the chemotherapy drugs that are approved for use by the FDA. Many people travel halfway across the country to seek attention from a highly regarded oncologist or participate in a clinical trial that holds more hope of survival by using a cutting-edge therapy. To do this, most people have to confront major logistical problems, including cost, lodging, and health insurance coverage. Our family was no different in this regard, except that we had an extra constraint: our young children.

For his medical care, Randy was debating between the standard regimen offered at the University of Pittsburgh and an experimental program offered in Seattle, Washington, and Houston, Texas. The clinical trial differed from the standard treatment by using three chemotherapy drugs that had shown promise in killing pancreatic cancer cells, along with daily radiation sessions to kill the cells as they tried to divide and replicate. Early results showed a 40 percent survival rate for the first year in a study group of one hundred people. When Randy compared the clinical trial's 40 percent one-year survival rate to the standard of care's 20 percent one-year survival rate, he immediately picked the clinical trial. There was a downside, though: horrendous side effects, such as reduced white blood cell count, extreme weight loss, diarrhea, fatigue, nausea, and even death. One of his Pittsburgh oncologists warned him not to subject himself to such a brutal regimen, but I remember Randy saying he wanted the oncologists to throw the kitchen sink at him. Then, if the cancer came back, he would have no regrets because he would have tried his hardest. The Houston-based program accepted Randy as a candidate for its clinical trial, allowing him to be a little closer to the East Coast, just a short flight away from Pittsburgh. However, the trade-off for greater survival rates also increased the level of complication for our family.

In my naïveté, I still hadn't wrapped my head around what this location choice meant to us as a family or to me as a mother and wife. I didn't have the knowledge or experience to understand how debilitating chemotherapy and radiation is to the body, how sick it makes the patient, or how weak that person becomes after being on a cancer regimen for a period of time. The oncologists understood what would happen to Randy's body during two months of treatment and strongly recommended that he bring a full-time caregiver to help manage the side effects from the treatment's high toxicity. I was shocked when Randy asked me to be his caregiver. I remember thinking, *How can I be in Houston taking care of Randy and in Pittsburgh taking care of our children?* I talked to Randy about having friends and family be with him during the week and I would fly down on the weekends. But he was adamant; he wanted only me to be his primary caregiver. At that moment, I felt he was being selfish and unfair to me. Thinking about it now, I can only surmise that Randy trusted me to see him get weaker and loved me enough to let his guard down. I think this is the nature of a strong marriage: one can be completely vulnerable with one's spouse, knowing that person is going to act with one's best intentions in mind. Knowing the punishment he was soon to undergo, my husband knew he could be sick, have terrible diarrhea, nausea, weight loss, lack of patience, and other reactions, and I would still love him. I guess I was a safe haven for him. He had seen me care for the children. He knew I would help him at all costs. The price of leaving my children, though, was high, maybe too high.

Rather than reject his request immediately, I struggled to find an acceptable alternative. The simple answer to me was to move the whole family to Houston, where we could be together and I could care for both Randy and the children, with additional help, of course. My solution turned out to be a total impossibility. Randy was an excellent time manager and could see how the idea would never work. He tried to dissuade me, but I needed to investigate the possibility and find the answer myself. I couldn't accept splitting up our family so quickly.

In October 2006, we visited the Houston cancer center, with five-month-old Chloe in tow, for preliminary tests. At that point, I realized that cancer centers are not family-friendly settings. In fact, there were some hospital floors and departments that Randy would need to go to where children were not allowed. Another problem would have been integrating the children's schedule with medical appointments. Most of us have experienced a long wait in a doctor's office. Cancer centers are no different. We found that Randy's appointment times were more like suggestions. We often waited long past the designated hour to receive a treatment or see the oncologist. Many services, such as cleaning intravenous lines used to administer chemotherapy, were on a first-come–first-served basis. I wondered to myself how I would arrange a predictable schedule to care for both Randy and the children. A nursing infant requires regular feedings, but I couldn't guarantee I would be there for Chloe when she was hungry or if she got hungry before her scheduled feeding. It would be a logistical nightmare. If I pursued this idea of bringing the children with us, I would be setting up a difficult situation from which we would all suffer.

After our initial trip in October 2006, I understood that Dylan, Logan, and Chloe couldn't be with us for those two difficult months, November and December 2006. My heart broke at the thought of being separated from my little ones, especially the baby. I cried and cried as I agonized over the decision to accompany Randy or abandon him for our children. How does one make this choice? My decision would have enormous repercussions for everyone in our family and especially on my marriage. As with any difficult decision, it's best to take time, think things through, and stay rational. I know my emotions tend to take over. So given my disposition, I took the time to think through the various aspects, to give voice to my feelings and concerns, and to share these thoughts with close friends. I asked questions of people who had been through the cancer caregiving experience. Several of our church friends had taken care of loved ones or had witnessed family members going through cancer treatments and offered me insights from their experiences and observations. They would approach me after the service or call me at home to talk with me. Our nanny, Amy, shared with me how her uncle and father-in-law benefited greatly by having their spouses with them during their battles with cancer.

In addition to talking with friends, I tried to frame the question of what to do in a helpful way. I asked myself: In five years, would my children remember or be scarred by my absence for two months? Would switching Chloe to formula hurt her? My answer was no to both these questions. Then I thought about Randy: Would my presence benefit him during the cancer treatment? Would I make a difference and potentially help him beat the cancer? I believed I could make a big difference in helping him at this time. Having thought through the pros and cons carefully and having given myself the time to articulate them gave me complete peace of mind as I went to my husband and our family. I told them our plan was for me to go with Randy to Houston. I found I would repeat this decision-making process over and over throughout his illness, and I still find it useful today. I try not to act impulsively, but rather take a step back and look at both the emotional and intellectual reactions I have, seek out additional information, and then make the best decision I can. In that way, I am less likely to feel regret over the path I choose.

Family and friends stepped up to help us by offering to care for the children while we were in Houston. Ultimately my older brother, Bob, and his wife, Jane, carved out space in their three-bedroom house. My thirteen-year-old nephew, Jacob, gave up his bedroom and slept on an air mattress in a room over the garage. Dylan took Jacob's bed, and Chloe slept in a borrowed crib, which took up most of the floor space. Eleven-year-old Hannah shared her room with Logan, who slept in another borrowed crib in the middle of the room. Even though I knew my little ones would be loved and well cared for, it was still painful to prepare them for this separation. Maybe when they were older the children wouldn't remember the time I was away from them, but in the moment, we were all feeling sad and heartbroken. I tried to explain to Dylan and Logan that I had to take care of their daddy, who was at a hospital far away, and I would be back every weekend to be with them. I tried to assure them I would always come back. Chloe was almost six months old when I nursed her for the last time, sitting in Bob and Jane's kitchen on Sunday, November 5, 2006. I handed my sister-in-law my baby, kissed the boys, and with promises I would return soon, I turned and walked out the door for the airport. I didn't cry in front of them, but waited until I was out of their sight to give free rein to the tears I had been holding back. My gut ached all the way to Houston until I was back with Randy and consumed once more by his needs.

This scene would play out seven more times, and in spite of my growing experience, each occasion felt more arduous than the last. Each time I tried to block out their cries of "Mommy, don't go!"

as I walked out the door but couldn't help melting into tears. My body was still making breast milk, so I'd have to pump to avoid becoming engorged and uncomfortable. Afterward I'd pour the milk down the drain mixed with tears of longing for my baby girl.

This shuttling between Randy and our children had to be one of the most difficult and stressful times of my entire life. I would spend the week in Houston caring for Randy as he grew weaker and as the pain and discomfort intensified. His treatments were administered in the hospital, then he would be released to recuperate in the hotel alone with me. I was frantic to help him but didn't really know how. I was sad and anxious much of the time. My life turned upside down. I was living in a hotel room and spending every waking hour fighting cancer Monday through Friday. I was woefully underprepared for my role as a cancer caregiver and for the medical and nursing responsibilities I was asked and expected to perform. No cancer center or oncology ward handed me a copy of a "What to Expect When You're a Caregiver" handbook—it doesn't exist. One learns as quickly as one can, in the moment. There isn't time to process the event, to allow one's feelings to settle, to wrap the mind around all that is happening. I didn't have a social worker or nurse to explain to me not only what Randy would be going through and the misery he would suffer mentally and physically, but also the shock I would experience at seeing my beloved suffer so greatly. Without this guidance, I walked blindly along, feeling my way and doing the best I could. Cancer centers and oncologists rely on caregivers, i.e., nonmedical help like me, to watch over the patient after leaving the oncologist's office. After a chemo session, a patient isn't held for observation but is released to go home. Some people don't have a lot of difficulties with their treatment. Others do, especially with a highly toxic drug taken over a long period of time. Chemo accumulates in the body, and its effects get stronger with each session. It seems kind of ironic that a person can be given these kinds of drugs and then immediately be released to go home, whereas when I got the flu shot this fall, I had to remain in the drugstore for thirty minutes to make sure I didn't have a reaction.

Once the patient leaves the oncologist's office, the burden is on the caregiver to observe and help with side effects from chemotherapy or radiation or disease progression. Some of the warning signs I was told to look for were:

fever

water retention

not urinating

decrease or increase in appetite

decrease or increase in weight

fatigue

pain

redness or inflammation around the port or peripherally inserted central catheter (PICC) line to administer chemotherapy or fluids

diarrhea

high or low blood pressure

To miss some of these changes in Randy's health could allow for serious problems to crop up or jeopardize his life. If Randy started to retain water, for example, I could tell by pressing on his shins. If my fingers left red marks, that meant fluid was building up. Water retention, or edema, would be a sign his kidneys were not working well due to the chemotherapy drugs, which can lead to kidney failure. That's bad! I felt a lot of pressure to watch over my husband. He wasn't just a patient to me, and I couldn't treat his suffering at arm's length. When he was in pain, it pained me. When he was uncomfortable, I felt discomfort. I once heard a palliative doctor say that one of the most difficult things the family goes through is watching their loved one live with pain and discomfort caused by cancer and its treatments. I heartily agree.

Caregiving really pushed me to grow in ways I never expected I could. I didn't believe I had it in me to take on the nursing responsibilities for Randy. One particularly difficult task I was asked to do was to clean and flush Randy's PICC line. This responsibility began in Houston and went on until Randy finished the chemotherapy regimen six months later. A PICC line is a thin plastic tube that's inserted into a vein, in the forearm in Randy's case, and is pushed up and up until it gets to a larger vein closer to the heart. The catheter is connected to the forearm skin by a little plastic wing held in place by three ugly, fragile, black sutures. The catheter allows a nurse to inject a chemo drug without constantly sticking a needle into a vein over and over again.

Veins become a big deal when a person undergoes chemo treatment for a long period of time. Cancer patients are often getting their veins punctured for blood tests or used as a conduit for fluids, like chemo drugs. After a while, those veins get overused and are prone to collapse or scarring, which means they are no longer usable for injections. Nurses search for a good vein, looking at arms, hands and even feet, much to the discomfort of the patient. Chemotherapy causes the veins to shrink, making it difficult for a nurse to find a vein and painful for the patient who gets poked over and over. Randy and I wanted to avoid this particular experience, so the PICC line was the best option.

There was a lot riding on keeping the PICC line free of infections or clogs. Randy needed the line to stay in excellent working order so he could do continuous chemotherapy to complete the protocol that he believed gave him the best chance to beat the cancer. There's nothing like a little pressure for proper motivation. In November 2006, my training began by watching a teaching video of the cleaning and flushing procedure of a PICC line on a real human arm. I think the video lasted about fifteen minutes, maybe a little bit more. During that infernally long time, I squirmed a hole into the bottom of my chair. I remember feeling nauseated, breaking out in a cold sweat, and averting my eyes from the video. I was horrified that I was going to have to take off the sterile bandaging from Randy's hairy forearms, pulling the hair and skin. Then I'd have to rub alcohol all around the area, including under the plastic wings and around the sutures. Ugh! My mind and stomach rebelled against the idea of touching a Q-tip to those stitches!

Randy was upset and frustrated with my reaction. He worried that he would have to make extra trips to the hospital to have a nurse clean his PICC line, costing him valuable energy and time, plus another medical visit on top of the countless other oncology, radiation, chemo, and scans he was scheduled regularly to do. I, in turn, became frustrated with his lack of patience or empathy for me and my feelings. Didn't it matter that I was pushing myself to tackle something that caused me so much discomfort? Couldn't I have a moment to be human and weak? I didn't go to nursing or medical school. I didn't even stay a candy striper for more than a year because the sights and smells in the hospital made me feel sick to my stomach. Didn't it say something about my dedication and love for him that I was willing to focus on the task at hand and ignore the smell and sight of the threads pulled through and knotted in human skin? Randy's disappointment and his impatience with my imperfections as a caregiver cut me deeply and caused a lot of strife in our relationship. The resentment we felt at this time started to build. We didn't talk to each other about what we were feeling, letting those negative feelings fester inside.

Even under watchful, caring eyes, Randy was becoming haggard, edgy, and exhausted. I'd never seen someone I loved so sick, and it took a toll on me to watch him get sicker as each day, each week passed. Taking a shower was now a major event for which Randy would have to muster his energy. The distance from the hotel room to the hospital across the street became a demanding walk. At the beginning, it would take us five minutes to reach most hospital locations, but as the weeks passed, it would take fifteen to thirty minutes. Randy refused to use a wheelchair, and we would walk slowly, stopping often for him to rest. He would put his hands on his hips, bend over slightly, and grimace in an expression of pain that would send chills up my spine. I could only encourage him and offer him my support, which I felt was not enough for him in his condition. I felt helpless, frustrated, and scared as his health declined more and more. Even though he felt miserable, as though he had the flu during those two months, Randy didn't complain or feel sorry for himself. Yes, he could be irritable, but he really tried not to lash out at those around him. When Randy's best friend since eighth grade, Jack Sheriff, came to take care of him on a couple of weekends, he noted that Randy seemed to disconnect from the emotional and focus on the scientific aspects of the situation. To divert himself, he would work on his computer, communicating with his research team and his colleagues. We would watch NFL football, and he would school me in the rules of the game if he had the energy. Early in the treatment, Jack took him to a sports bar and noticed that Randy seemed relieved to be among "normal" people who were out living their lives. He was removed from the cancer world and could forget about what his new normal was, even if it was for just a couple of hours. Most of the time, though, he slept or sat quietly.

After a Whipple procedure, it's normal for people to go through a difficult period of getting their digestive tract to work properly again. Randy was no different. His body was not happy with its new arrangement and complained bitterly by refusing to digest food and instead sending it on its way to his colon. Randy and I struggled to find foods and portion sizes that he could manage. Sugary, fatty, or spicy foods were intolerable. Later, when undergoing the clinical trial program of chemotherapy and radiation, Randy experienced a further reduction in diet because his system was so stressed. Radiation burns off the cilia inside the intestines, creating a unique condition called slick gut, so named because food slides through without any nutrition being extracted. Chemotherapy drugs' side effects often include nausea and diarrhea, which further reduce a person's caloric intake.

Getting calories into Randy became a major priority for us. For breakfast, he could usually eat a scrambled egg, but it had to be hot out of the pan. Randy would sometimes get up for breakfast around ten or eleven, or earlier to make a doctor's appointment. When we were living in the hotel room in Houston, I bought a hot plate and some cheap pans to cook for Randy. But a hot plate can't cook things very quickly. So when Randy would say, "I think I could eat a plate of plain spaghetti," I would jump up and start cooking. Unfortunately, by the time I would have his food ready, the craving would have passed; he would take one bite and sadly shake his head. A little while later, he would say, "I think I could eat some tomato soup." I'd quickly make him soup and served him in bed, only to have him eat a spoonful or two and then refuse the rest of it. At other times, I'd go downstairs to the hotel cantina to get the soda or juice he was craving. Or I'd walk over to the cancer center's cafeteria for something for which he expressed a desire to eat and that I couldn't make in the room. Sometimes he would still want to eat it by the time I got back, sometimes not. This scenario would repeat itself many times over the course of Randy's battle, whether in the hospital or at home.

The evidence of my failed attempts to whet Randy's appetite were quantifiable from the several boxes of nonperishable foods Randy had started off liking and then stopped as treatments progressed. After those few months in Houston, I was well trained to jump whenever Randy said he was hungry. As his weight dropped and the threat of stopping treatment increased, I felt more and more frantic, more like a failure, as though I had let him down. Somehow in my irrational mind, I was responsible for Randy's weight loss or gain, for finding something that would tempt him to take even a few bites. Randy didn't complain to me or blame me. But the sadness and the pain in his eyes were unmistakable.

I turned to the hospital nutritionist for advice; she had years of experience working with cancer patients who had faced the same challenges. She had a wealth of information and tricks to get the calories in, and a lot of them worked. The program coordinator and oncologist also were very helpful in addressing the chemo side effects. In addition to an over-the-counter antidiarrheal medication taken every four hours, they recommended adding a prescription antidiarrheal medication. Even with doses every two hours, Randy's diarrhea continued at a dangerous rate. The next step was to add tincture of opium to the arsenal. Thank you, Blue Cross Blue Shield, for approving the prescription, because adding this third medication was the charm. Randy was able to stabilize his weight, and I breathed a sigh of relief. By the time he finished the treatment's eight-week regimen, Randy had dropped 35 pounds and weighed around 147. His six-foot frame looked emaciated, but he had completed the treatment protocol without interruption. The odds were looking good for now.

I don't recall Randy saying he missed the children during the time he spent in Houston, most likely because he had steeled himself to the separation. Plus, he believed that the sacrifice he made now would pay off by killing all the cancer and allowing him to be there with them as they grew up. He could keep the long-term goal in the forefront of his mind and not be distracted by the short-term pain. But I'm sure the children were never far from his thoughts. Our nanny, Amy, had made us a beautiful photo album of the children to take with us, and we flipped through it many times.

After the draining week in Houston caring for Randy, I would hop on a plane to spend a hectic and emotional weekend in Virginia with our children. Instead of our time together being some idyllic Hollywood scene where each moment was precious and perfect, I struggled to switch gears and parent three small children without any help. I'd been raised half my life in this small town, spending many summers at my grandparents' house. Now as an adult I found myself lost in this little town. I didn't know how to drive to places I'd been to as a child. I didn't know what kind of child-friendly outings were available. To compound matters, I didn't have time or energy to look up things to do with the children during the time we were together. So I'd find myself worrying about how to manage their energy and have a meaningful and magical visit with them.

Our routine went something like this: after getting in from the airport late on Friday night, I'd pick up the children at my brother's house Saturday morning, around eight a.m. The first Saturday I came by, the children were still in pajamas, but by the end of the two months, Bob and Jane would be standing in the driveway with the kids and weekend bags ready to go, a telltale sign that this arrangement was taking its toll on them as well. We'd stop by the grocery store together to pick up milk and something for dinner, then drive the two miles down the road to my parents' three-bedroom house. My mother was usually gone during the day, taking care of her elderly parents at their house. My father was working in Richmond, Virginia. So it was just the four of us out in the country, in the peace and calm—or rather in isolation, which is how I saw it. My parents live off a busy two-lane country road lined by deep ditches that could swallow a car. With no other children to play with and nothing to walk to, we made our own fun.

Virginia has a mild winter compared to Pittsburgh: blue skies, highs in the fifties. Dylan and Logan could run around in the backyard while I held Chloe. Still, it was hard to find a rhythm like the one we had in Pittsburgh at our home. I felt off-kilter, unsure of what to do or where we could go. I'm embarrassed to say I felt overwhelmed, low on both physical and emotional energy. How could I feel that way when I missed them all week? When I loved being a mother and hanging out with my children? To compound my feelings of inadequacy, Chloe wouldn't take a bottle from me. I was still lactating and she could smell the milk. She'd lie in my arms crying hungrily but rejecting the formula I was offering her.

I couldn't nurse her because if I did, she wouldn't take the bottle during the week, and that would make life difficult for everyone. Finally, her pathetic cries wore me down, and I called my sister-in-law to come over to get Chloe to eat. This scenario surely wasn't part of my romanticized dreams of what the time with my children should be like. The pressure I placed on myself and the expectations of a perfect family time were more than I could live up to, and it brought me down, down, down.

Even though staying around my parents' house was the easiest thing to do, it was boring—at least I thought the children would be bored. No toys, no crafts, no tricycles, no nothing like we had at home. Dylan and Logan didn't ask for anything but to be together with me. It was I who had set these expectations of maintaining our normal, precancer lifestyles in an unfamiliar setting. Since the children woke up around six a.m. each morning, we had plenty of daylight hours to fill before bedtime at eight p.m. Often we'd explore the outdoors in the early morning. Then we'd go somewhere else for a change of scenery and an adventure. Now anytime we went somewhere it was like troop movements. I was weighed down with the baby in a carrier on the front, diaper bag with snacks and formula hanging from one arm, and two little hands holding mine. Just keeping up with the boys with a baby attached to my body took a lot of energy.

Once we went to the Children's Museum of Virginia in Portsmouth (about thirty minutes away), and the boys enjoyed the various hands-on exhibits while Chloe enjoyed the toddler's area. Another time we found a playground close to my grandmother's house. One rainy Saturday, I took them to McDonald's for lunch and to play in the play area. It seemed like an easy adventure until Logan lifted his open milk container to his mouth and soaked his clothes, the table, and the floor. I could see the accident happen before it actually did, but I couldn't intervene because I had the baby laid in one arm while feeding her with my free hand. It all seems so innocent, so simple a problem, but at the time, the incident was magnified out of proportion. My nerves and my psyche were raw, and the littlest things seemed to draw blood. I gave Logan my most disappointed-in-you look, yelled for the boys to get their shoes on, and stomped out the door with two sad little boys in tow.

I struggled to manage the everyday, normal demands of child rearing. I hadn't learned to make things as simple as possible, like buying prepared meals at the grocery store or picking up takeout because there was limited food delivery in our area. Even after an exhausting day, I would push myself harder. For dinner, I cooked and then had to clean up the kitchen while trying to supervise the children. Chloe would sit in her bouncy seat or ExerSaucer while her brothers watched a cartoon on television. Afterward, I still had to give the children baths and supervise brushing teeth—activities that demanded still more energy. After baths and pajamas, the boys would pick out a book, and I'd read to each of them. The boys slept in one room: Dylan in the single bed, Logan in the crib. Chloe and I were in a room across the hall. Even though exhausted, I would still wake up every time the baby tossed and turned or made any noise, to see if all were fine. Then the sun would rise, and I would start another day sleep deprived.

The physical toll on me was apparent in the weight I gained during this period. But more visually striking and more painful was the eczema that flared up on my eyelids. Eczema is an inflammation of the skin that can be triggered by dry air, pollution, and stress. In my case, my eyelids were slightly swollen and the skin raw and painful. I couldn't wear eye makeup at all, but would slather on Vaseline to help protect the skin and calm the flare-up. The area would heal and the skin would become scaly and flake, only to erupt again, and the process would repeat itself. I remember Randy asking his oncologist if there was a medication he could prescribe to give me some relief, since we were thousands of miles away from our family doctor. He refused, saying I wasn't his patient and I would need to contact a local dermatologist. As it usually takes six months to get an appointment with a dermatologist, I simply lived with the annoyance.

Regular exercise also took a back burner, but I got on the treadmill whenever I could. I tried to take the stairs instead of the elevator or escalator at the hospital. And on rare occasions, I would take a fast walk outside in the mild Houston fall weather. I was used to exercising at the gym twice a week, taking a yoga class once a week, and playing with the children. Pittsburgh is also a walking city where I would push the stroller to the library, playground, coffee shop, and even grocery store. In Houston, I didn't have those built-in opportunities for daily activity.

For now, my energies were dedicated to my loved ones. They were my top priorities; my needs would wait. But it was a difficult balancing act, one in which I felt I could never please everyone. At the end of the day, I had to accept that I could only do my best; that would have to be good enough. Right now it was easier to separate Randy's needs from the children's. I could also dedicate myself completely to either when I was with them because they were physically separated. The real test came when we were back together in Pittsburgh after Randy finished his treatment in Houston. Then I would have to prioritize in real time with real and long-lasting consequences accompanying each choice.

5

Help! I'm in Over My Head

THERE'S A PIVOTAL SCENE in *An Officer and a Gentleman* where Lou Gossett Jr.'s character, Gunnery Sergeant Foley, breaks Richard Gere's cocky, emotionally walled-off officer candidate character, Zack Mayo, by putting him through grueling workout after workout until Mayo finally can't take any more. He can't be an island unto himself, and he accepts the fact that he must change to grow as a person and to become a team player. He learns that being strong doesn't mean doing everything oneself or that opening oneself up to love and expressing that love isn't a form of weakness.

During my time as a caregiver, I came to identify with Zack Mayo. But instead of a hunky Lou Gossett Jr., life and cancer played the part of my drill sergeants, placing one burden after another on my shoulders. The load got heavier and heavier, and though I was stooped over with my back breaking, I kept telling myself I could carry on without imposing on other people or accepting their help.

I continued to mother Dylan, Logan, and Chloe and do all of the same activities, like taking them to the zoo and to the natural history museum. In my mind, I didn't see time or my energies as part of a zero-sum game, so my intention to give the children the same amount of time while adding the tremendously consuming job of caregiver to my plate didn't seem unreasonable. I knew it would be a juggling act, but I figured I would be perfectly able to nurse and care for Randy in Pittsburgh as I had been doing in Houston, even with the addition of the children tied to my apron strings.

Despite the help we had with the children during the day, I wasn't doing a good job of dividing my time between them and Randy. Nor was I getting enough rest. The perfect schedule would have been to spend early morning hours with the children, midday with Randy, put the children down for their naps in the early afternoon, late afternoon with Randy again, cook dinner, and then resume care of the children until bedtime. Even being conscious of my time allocation, there were always variations in daily events—visits to the oncologist, children's holiday parties, doctor appointments, or someone being sick. Looking back now, I can see I was on a collision course with reality. The paradox I missed at the time was that my efforts to care for my children and husband would be undone by exhaustion. My mistake was trying to live my life as it had been before cancer. The way I approached every aspect of my normal life would have to change dramatically.

Life sent me a serious wake-up call about the mess I was making. After four months of unrelenting giving, I finally hit rock bottom. It was a cold Friday in February 2007. Randy was on a 5-FU (fluorouracil) chemotherapy regimen via drip infusion. Some people experience mild side effects, but he was having a tough time with diarrhea and fatigue, along with reduced appetite. A minor cosmetic result of chemotherapy was that his hair turned a coarse wiry gray. He rested in bed in the back bedroom during the day and in the basement at night. With his white blood cell count low and weight down to around 140 pounds, Randy couldn't tolerate the cold, so we kept a space heater nearby to keep the room at 80 degrees. That particular Friday was no different from most. Logan and Dylan went to preschool in the morning, and Chloe was at home crawling about. As usual, I divided my time between the kids and Randy with the help of Amy and our babysitter, Laura O'Malley. Then at around ten o'clock that evening, something completely normal but utterly devastating to our fragile balance occurred. Dylan woke up with a terrible bout of stomach flu. Families go through this all the time. But in our case, Randy's susceptibility to infection added a new dimension to the situation that I had not thought of or encountered before.

I had been in bed for only thirty minutes when I heard Dylan crying out for me. For the next several hours, I helped him to the bathroom, holding his head over the toilet or cleaning him up after an accident. Around one in the morning, Chloe woke up crying for her bottle. But I couldn't go to her. Dylan was still vomiting. He needed me most, and I knew she wouldn't die if she missed one feeding. Still, the guilt welled up inside me. Then Randy appeared and offered to give Chloe her bottle. He had been asleep in the basement while all this was going on, so I was surprised to see him. After the baby was fed, he went back down to sleep in the basement, and I continued to care for Dylan. By four a.m., I was exhausted. I hadn't slept all night and had been busy the previous day. I went down to the basement and asked Randy if he would watch over Dylan for an hour so I could get a little sleep before the other two children woke up. There wouldn't be a sitter coming on Saturday, and I would have to care for the baby and our energetic toddler along with Dylan.

I was blindsided by Randy's reaction. He was furious at me for not taking care of myself during the day in case I had to handle an all-nighter by myself. In his weakened state, the flu could kill him, he said. Here he had subjected himself to surgery and a painful two-month regimen in order to give himself the best chances of surviving, and I was jeopardizing his odds by asking him to take care of Dylan. In that moment, I felt just awful, like a failure for not being able to juggle everything by myself, for having to ask Randy for help when he was so ill, for not being better prepared for inevitable moments like sick children, for not having a backup plan. This is what it's going to be like when I'm a single parent, I thought, so I might as well get used to it. It became crystal clear to me in this moment that I had to change my mind-set. We weren't a normal two-parent family anymore, and I couldn't fall back on Randy for help. I needed outside help, and I had to ask for it, fast.

At six in the morning, I called my next-door neighbor, who I knew was an early riser. I explained what was happening and asked her to please come over. Then I sent out e-mails to all my friends and sitters, asking if someone could help with the children that day. A new morning, a new beginning, a new strategy. I started acting like a manager, delegating responsibilities and doing the things only I could do. Even though I accepted this direction as the best for me, the children, and Randy, my conscience was at war with itself.

In my mind, it was my responsibility as wife and mother to be tireless in caring for the children and Randy. Moreover, I was raised to be self-sufficient, independent. Not meeting my family's demands and accepting help from others would mean I was a failure.

I also didn't want to be an arms-length mother! I wanted to be directly involved in their lives, putting Band-Aids on boo-boos and going to play dates with them. I didn't want to let go of my old life, the way things were, and accept what the circumstances of the moment dictated. I felt as if I was being buffeted about in a tumultuous sea where the waves were crashing over my head and no land was in sight. Of course it didn't occur to me that I was being an even worse mother and wife by wearing myself down and taking it all on the chin.

I also imagined that this was for only a short period of time in the grand scheme of things. It wouldn't always be like this. I would be able to go back and assume the reins again. But poor Randy! He could see the big picture long before I could; he just couldn't get me up to speed. He was so frustrated with me, so disappointed that I hadn't adjusted more quickly to our changing family dynamics. And he felt abandoned by me because my attention was divided. I was not as focused on him or his fight to beat the cancer as I needed to be. This was not a new issue in our relationship, but rather one we had worked through many times since the arrival of children. How I divided my time between the children and Randy was a dilemma more emphasized by Randy's illness. In addition, Randy prided himself on his time-management skills, so he could be quick to criticize how others managed their time. He believed in using time wisely and efficiently and often gave talks on the subject. He was so tuned in to how he used his time at work that he would keep an electronic log of how many minutes he spent on certain tasks, then he would evaluate the data and decide how he could work more productively. Because he did this exercise for his own time, he felt others could and should do it for theirs. I hadn't truly embraced that approach in my personal life, and Randy was critical of how I chose to allocate my energies. He was a very smart man who trusted his intellect and his ability to make sound decisions in any given situation. I wasn't as smart or as quick as he was, and I think it tried his patience—not that he loved me any less, but I think he felt he could make decisions better than I. In the past, I had often pointed out to him that if he made decisions for other people, then it wouldn't be their lives they were living. Not being the best time manager or having a backup plan for illnesses might not seem dire in a normal circumstance, but it played out as a complete disaster in Randy's mind. As a compromise, I agreed to rearrange my daily schedule to allow more rest for me and to go to bed at an earlier hour.

However, there was a bigger life lesson than time management for me. From the stomach flu episode, I came to understand that being strong doesn't mean not asking for help, nor does it mean not being scared. This is probably one of the greatest lessons I've ever received. I needed to offload some of my responsibilities and free myself a little to manage the load better. I had to admit that I could no longer be the same kind of mother I had been when Dylan was little; it wasn't possible. I could not be with the kids *and* be with Randy in the oncology wards. I had to ask for help—and lots of it. I couldn't cook dinner every night from scratch using fresh vegetables from the farmer's market, so I gratefully accepted dinners of any kind from the families at my sons' preschool. I don't know if they used organic produce, and I learned not to give it a thought. I ordered take-out dinners using a gift card generously provided by my husband's colleagues at Carnegie Mellon University. I even took people up on their offer to unpack my family's possessions—yes, even my clothes and underwear—to get us back into our newly renovated house in Pittsburgh. Was I a lesser mom, wife, and woman for this? No! In fact, it made our lives better to let others pitch in. I had more energy to devote to all of those around me; I wasn't so stressed out and grouchy. It made life seem more manageable, which in turn lightened my mood.

I not only had to accept the idea of help from others, but I also had to come to terms with people being in our house more often and on a more intimate footing than normal. I had no problem with friends and neighbors helping to unpack our sheets, towels, or children's clothes, but when it came to my things, someone putting my clothes in the closet or in the drawer made me feel uncomfortable even though I knew it was saving me valuable time and energy. I also happened to overhear my neighbors commenting on our laundry room setup; we had two sets of washers and dryers. I wanted to go in and explain how one of the washers was from my grandmother, who no longer could operate it due to dementia, and the second dryer was an old one left in the house by the previous owners. I felt I had to justify our choices by explaining how Randy had thought it would be good time management to have a second set because we were so often washing sheets and children's clothes. But I didn't say anything to them; I quietly walked away. I didn't feel I should be scrutinized, nor should I have to justify anything. I didn't want my lifestyle exposed or to be judged for how we had chosen to set up our house or anything else. My life felt very transparent, very public, but I didn't feel I had the right to complain, since we needed the help so desperately. I kept telling myself this was a small price to pay and to be grateful. Randy didn't seem bothered in the least by people's presence in our house or their handling our more intimate things. He was never very attached to things, nor did he pay any mind to what other people said. Moreover, he got to stay ensconced in his office working on his computer while I managed the logistics.

So he was not only mentally distant from the goings-on, but also physically distant as well.

Looking back, asking for help sounds reasonable. But it was an emotionally charged issue for me and a hard lesson for me to learn. Even when I agreed to accept help, I still had to get my head in a good place about receiving it. I had to change not only myself but my image of myself in order to find peace. Finally, I had to accept that asking for help is a sign of intelligence and strength. When you are in difficult straits, identifying the areas where you need an extra hand or a smarter brain takes honesty and courage.

When people say to me now, "I don't know how you did it," I proudly respond, "With a lot of help from a lot of wonderful people." Many of our friends and family seemed to know intuitively how to help. They would see something that needed to be done, do it, and then ask permission later. It could be as simple as starting some laundry or cleaning up the kitchen. I loved it when people gave me lists of specific tasks they could do for me. I appreciated not having to expend energy generating a to-do list of my own. I've been asked repeatedly by folks who want to help a friend or relative who is a caregiver what they can do to make a difference. My answer is: everyday tasks like housekeeping, grocery shopping, fixing dinner, or doing the laundry. I also found that friends coming over to sit with Randy, talk with him, massage his back, or watch television with him gave me great peace of mind and gave Randy the companionship he needed.

But there's a fine line between being helpful and imposing. There were times when I'd had a terrible day and I'd want a little down-time to decompress, to sit quietly without anyone else around, without the obligation to be social—a time when I could loosen the stranglehold on my emotions. Sometimes, a well-intentioned friend would misread my mood as being one in which I needed a shoulder to cry on or an ear for listening. I would try to be polite and explain that I was tired and needed rest, but that person might not be using "listening ears," as preschool teachers like to say. She might insist on staying at our house until the dishwasher had finished running so she could put away the clean dishes, even after I had explained that what I really needed was to go to bed. Finally, I would leave my well-intentioned friend sitting by herself at the kitchen table while I went to find some solitude.

6

The Toll of Caregiving

EVEN WITH LOTS OF HELP from family and friends with the children, I still found myself exhausted by day's end. Every night I would be in bed by ten p.m., striving for eight hours of sleep, minus time feeding the baby and taking care of the boys during the night, if necessary. My body felt like a lead weight as I slipped gratefully under the covers and turned off the lights. But instead of falling into a deep and peaceful sleep, my brain continued to spin as I tossed and turned, trying to find a more comfortable position. Thoughts came relentlessly. Some were unusually outlandish worries, and they would fester and grow as I allowed myself to fall down that black hole of "What if . . ."

One particular internal dialogue went like this:

What am I going to do if there's a fire in the house? How am I going to get the children out safely? I'd mentally chew on it as I lay in bed by myself with the children asleep down the hall and Randy ensconced in his basement retreat.

Which child should I go to first?

Maybe Dylan—he's the oldest and the most self-sufficient.

But how am I going to get him from the second floor to the ground without him getting hurt?

I pored over the possibilities. My mind continued to whir.

I know. I'll tie the bed sheets together, tie one end around his waist, and lower him to the ground. Then he can run next door and get help.

What about Logan? He's only two years old. Would he be able to get down the same way?

Yes, this should work for him, too.

Without pause, my thoughts moved right to Chloe: *I think I could lower the baby to the ground.*

OK, now I've solved the problem if a fire breaks out downstairs. Great! Now I can rest easy. I can sleep.

But no, my synapses continued to hum: *What if the fire starts upstairs? And what about Randy in the basement?* The moon would slowly move across the nighttime sky while I worked through ever more scenarios, trying to contemplate what seemed to me plausible threats to our family. Bad things happen to people, and now I had learned we were vulnerable, living in a hostile world that didn't care how young Randy was, nor that he took care of himself, nor that we had three young children. Nothing shielded us from being one of those families one reads about in the newspaper or sees on a television show and one thinks, "There but for the grace of God go I!" Having just experienced two of the worst months of my entire life, I knew all too clearly how catastrophe could tear your world apart. I wanted to be prepared for the next time. I didn't want to be blindsided once more, as we had been when Randy was first diagnosed with pancreatic cancer. Though it was unreasonable to think I could plan for all possible challenges before they arose, I still tried—an attempt to feel that I had some control over my life. Cancer had left me feeling so vulnerable. My response was to create a sense of mastery over events in my life.

I wish I could have been lying next to my husband, turning to him to help me through these sleepless times. I had so many wonderful things to appreciate, to celebrate with him—how our family was growing, how we had remodeled our house to accommodate that growth, and how beautiful the moon was on these wintry nights. Together we had put so much thought and energy into the house project. This was our dream home, where we were to raise our family and where Randy and I planned to live until the children were grown and Randy retired from the university.

But Randy and I were in some ways worlds apart now. Instead of sleeping upstairs in our master bedroom with its beautiful windows looking out over the amazingly large city backyard, Randy was sleeping in the basement with the heat jacked up. The physical distance between the two of us translated into an emotional one. I was constantly tired from wearing so many hats—caregiver, mother, and house manager. I woke with Chloe at around one a.m. to give her a bottle, and then I was back up at six a.m. when the two boys were ready to start the day. I felt as if Randy didn't appreciate all that I was doing and how hard I was trying. For his part, he believed I wasn't spending enough time with him, that I was afraid to sit with him and be near the sick guy. Our wounded feelings festered until a couple of our friends suggested we see a counselor. They went so far as to argue that if Randy survived the cancer, our marriage might not. But we didn't need a marriage counselor; we needed someone who knew how to help people dealing with life-threatening illness and all the chaos and stress it could bring.

During a visit to our local Pittsburgh oncologist, Randy asked for

a recommendation for someone we could talk to who had experience with people in our situation. The oncologist knew of a psychotherapist who worked with cancer patients and their families.
And that's how we met one of the most wonderful, kind, insightful,
and intelligent people I have ever met: Dr. Michele Reiss. We were
fortunate to find a local practitioner who focused on mental issues
that arise in battling cancer.

From the first time we started talking with Dr. Reiss, she became an integral part of our cancer team. Whereas the oncologist
and the platoon of other doctors focused on the physical aspects of
Randy's cancer—how to stop the disease from spreading, control
pain, monitor nutrition, and prolong life—Dr. Reiss's specialty as a
psychotherapist addressed the mental health issues. Stress is something we all experience, but in excess and over long periods of time,
stress has a profound effect on a person's mental and physical state.
More and more medical studies are studying the impact of stress on
both the cancer patient's and the caregiver's health. In particular,
caregiving stress has been found to increase the caregiver's susceptibility to infectious disease and depression. The caregiver is also
more likely to suffer premature aging, a measurable decrease in life
expectancy (some studies suggest between three and ten years), as
well as risks associated with sleep deprivation.* Who would have
thought that being a dutiful loved one would take years off your
own life or make you sick!

Because the risks associated with stress and the impact that caregiving has on the individual are now coming to light, I hope that
more oncology practices will shift their treatment paradigm to en-

---

*Take Care! Self-Care for the Family Caregiver, National Family Caregivers Association,
www.thefamilycaregiver.org, winter 2006.

compass more than just the physical aspects of cancer. Currently, many cancer centers and oncology groups maintain a wonderfully strong team of doctors, from radiologists to oncologists to surgeons. However, they neglect the psychological aspect the disease brings with it. Cancer specialists address nutrition and pain, yet they ignore how devastating it can be to live with cancer or face death as the disease spreads to other parts of the body. Moreover, medical science and technology have made significant strides in slowing or stopping cancer cells from multiplying. As a result, a patient often lives longer with the disease in remission. However, a person surviving longer with cancer or other illness presents a new set of challenges that need to be addressed. One of these is how to offer support to both patient and caregiver as they strive to not only live their lives, but maintain a quality of life. Counseling could help address some of the needs. Randy and I were proactive enough to find a therapist to help us, but others might not go that route and need to have the resource offered to them.

As Randy admitted in *The Last Lecture,* he was not a big fan of psychologists. But after working with Dr. Reiss, he understood the benefits: "Now, with my back against the wall, I see how hugely helpful [counseling] can be. I wish I could travel through oncology wards telling this to patients who are trying to tough it out on their own." Randy held very strong opinions, and it took a lot to get him to change his position on a subject. So it is a testament both to how much he suffered emotionally and to Dr. Reiss's exceptional abilities that Randy embraced therapy.

When we first stepped into Dr. Reiss's office, both Randy and I were feeling disappointed in each other. One of the first things she did was to have us listen to each other. I mean *really* listen to what the other person was saying. We realized that even though we were going through Randy's cancer together, our individual experiences were unique and valid. For his part, Randy experienced daily pain after the surgical procedure to remove the tumor, as well as terrible side effects from the chemotherapy. On the other hand, I was trying to maintain a normal routine for our three children, provide the best care I could for Randy, and manage our household. Randy communicated to me that he wanted to do everything he could to maximize his chances of living. To achieve this goal, he had to make the treatment and any additional options his highest priority. He would push his body as hard as he could by taking the highest chemotherapy dosages allowed, and he wanted my support for him during that time, regardless of what he looked like or how bad he felt. For my part, I explained to Randy that I felt I had to be the one who dealt with the issues of the moment, whether it was his feeling terrible and needing extra attention or filing our taxes or investigating kindergarten options for Dylan, who would start school in the upcoming fall. Our roles and points of view reminded me a lot of Virginia Woolf's *To the Lighthouse*. Mr. Ramsey can't see the red-hot poker flowers his wife admires growing around the house, but he can look up into the constellations and appreciate the stars, which she in turn cannot see. A similar dichotomy existed for Randy and me. Here we were a team, a united front, fighting pancreatic cancer to save his life. And yet we were coming from two different places that made it difficult to understand the other's commitment and contributions to the team effort. Listening to each other and respecting the different ways we were going through this experience helped bring us closer together. Our marriage stayed strong as we continued to walk this difficult path together.

Another issue Randy and I shared was stress-induced paralysis. We simply were unable to make a decision. This was most apparent in our need to choose a school for Dylan. Pittsburgh is a wonderful city that offers a full spectrum of educational options, both public and private. In the public sector, there are neighborhood schools, magnet schools, charter schools, and even an elementary school using the Montessori approach. On the other side of the coin are the independent schools offering traditional and nontraditional educations. Before Randy became ill, I had done a modicum of research into which setting would be best for Dylan. But since Randy's diagnosis, I had not been able to devote any time or energy into making a decision. Now in the spring of 2007, our window to enroll him was closing. We had to make a choice soon. After I had narrowed down the selection to just a few schools, Randy and I evaluated the options together, but we couldn't decide. So we visited the schools. Randy would unleash his sharp mind on the unsuspecting principal, who would be grilled for a good half hour. Randy would ask how the school would handle various scenarios, including what offense would have to be committed for a student to be kicked out of the school by the end of a school day, as well as questions about how the school allocated its funds. Even after gathering all this information, we still couldn't decide. Each question was preceded with the hypothetical, "If Randy should die of cancer . . ." Should we go with the private school located three houses away so I could easily walk Dylan to school with two little ones in tow? The magnet school might offer Dylan more educational enrichment opportunities, but it would be a longer bus commute. As the deadline loomed, our anxiety rose. During one of our sessions with Dr. Reiss, we explained our dilemma and asked her advice. Dr. Reiss showed us that we were allowing the stress and fear of living with cancer to prevent us from living our lives. Just as I would lie in bed at night working through every possible problem that might arise and how I would deal with it, Randy and I were doing the same thing with school choice. We were envisioning every possible scenario that we could think of, exhausting ourselves in the process, not realizing we could never conceive of every possibility.

Education wasn't the only decision we couldn't make. There were also little things, like whether or not to buy a rug for the front entryway. I would spin around and around asking myself if I should spend the money on a rug for a house we might have to leave if the cancer returned and Randy died. Randy, for his part, would complain of living with the Sword of Damocles hanging over his head. He felt that at any time the worst could happen. He wanted the two of us to decide in advance what we would do if the cancer returned. He talked about it with friends and family. He wanted to do everything he could to leave us in the best situation possible. So we talked about where the family should live—Pittsburgh or closer to my family? If we decided on my family, should that be closer to my older brother in Virginia or my younger brother in North Carolina? I wanted to remain in Pittsburgh, where I had a strong support network, good friends whom I cherish, and a real love for the city.

After listening to us, Dr. Reiss helped us learn another important lesson: cancer made us feel as if we had less control over our lives, and as a result, we were trying to exercise some dominion over the course of events. But we had to accept some loss of control and the inability to predict all outcomes or scenarios that would arise. Instead of spinning our wheels and agonizing over the what-ifs, we had to make the best decision we could at this moment with the information we had. Later on, we could reevaluate the decision we had made and make changes as new information or circumstances presented themselves.

Armed with this insight, Randy and I were able to go back and make the decisions we hadn't been able to before. We chose a school for Dylan. We decided not to decorate the newly renovated space. We even agreed on a strategy for where the family would live if Randy died. Then we filed the master plan away with the acknowledgment that we wouldn't discuss it further until absolutely necessary.

Having a counselor to talk to about the problems we encountered and the difficulties we had coping with them was a benefit to us beyond measure. It not only improved our daily lives in terms of making decisions, both big and small, but Randy and I were able to talk to each other and appreciate the other's point of view. Our relationship strengthened and our love flourished during a time of extraordinary duress. And it was a good thing, too, because we needed the foundation of our marriage to be rock solid so we could face even more demons on our cancer journey.

7

Cancer Blindsides Us Again

IT WAS A MAGICAL, GLORIOUS summer after so much stress
and work during the winter and spring of 2007. Randy was off
chemotherapy for the first time in six months, and he had re-
gained his weight and his vitality. We were living in the moment
without fear of what might happen tomorrow. Randy was so confident he was going to live that he got a new car to replace his worn-
out thirteen-year-old Volkswagen Cabriolet—the same one he had
poured Coke into while his niece and nephew watched with a mix-
ture of disbelief, humor, and horror. We took trips to Kennywood,
a Pittsburgh amusement park, and rode the rides with our children. Randy won a giant stuffed animal for the children, passing
on his love for carnival games and the thrill of walking through
the park with a humongous, orange clownfish for everyone to see.
We frequented the local water park, where Randy was courageous
enough to do the high body slide and some tubing with Dylan. We
vacationed for a week at the beach in the southern part of Virginia,

close to where my family lives, allowing us to visit my brother Bob
and his family again. Randy even felt strong enough for me to take
a nine-day trip to Spain with his mother, his sister, and her husband.
I was reluctant to go, but he insisted, saying he would have plenty of
help. He also felt that I needed a vacation. He really wanted me to
take this trip, I think, in part to allow him to do something for me.
I accepted and had a wonderful time and a much-needed break. Life
in the Pausch house was almost like old times.

At the end of summer, Randy was scheduled to return to Houston for a CT scan to see if the cancer cells had fought back and
begun multiplying again. In August 2007, Randy and I made our
travel plans but treated this trip as a romantic getaway for the two
of us to reconnect, building in some time to go to the hospital as
well as having a little side trip. Before seeing the oncologist to get
the results from Randy's scans, we traveled to Galveston Island to
experience one of the country's biggest indoor water parks: Schlitterbahn. Like amusement parks, water parks were high on our list
of fun activities. This visit to Schlitterbahn without children harked
back to the days when we were dating and first married, without
kids, when we would go to the local water park in Pittsburgh to
spend the day together riding all the slides. Seven years later in
Galveston, Texas, we were having the time of our lives. We tried
every slide in the seventy-thousand-square-foot park! Some were
very tall, and we had to climb flights of stairs after waiting in long
lines. Other slides were twisty and short. And of course there was
a long lazy river, which we floated down holding hands as though
we didn't have a care in the world. This excursion would not have
been possible just four months earlier, when Randy was so depleted
from chemotherapy. Instead, he was like his old self, like the Randy
I had first met and fallen in love with: energetic, upbeat, full of kid-

like excitement to try the next ride. It was a wonderful day, a sweet memory I treasure.

After such an upbeat experience, we walked into the oncologist's office in Houston full of confidence that the cancer had not returned. Nevertheless, we both experienced the usual "scanxiety"— the nervous feeling one gets at the approach of a scan date. Everyone who has ever had cancer feels anxious and a bit worried as a scan date approaches, even someone who has been cancer-free for ten years. Still, we felt pretty sure that Randy would dodge another bullet. How could he not? He looked and acted so healthy!

As we sat in the waiting area to see the oncologist, I remember looking around discreetly at the other couples and families. Statistically, someone sitting in that waiting room was going to hear bad news. I wondered who it might be. Usually when a patient and loved one would exit an examining room area crying softly, we collectively looked away while our hearts sank in our chests. I remember thinking that would not be us today. Not today. That's all I could hang my hat on.

Randy worked away on his laptop. I knew he was worried, but he kept it to himself. Then it was our turn. In a flash, Randy put away his laptop, slung his backpack onto his shoulder, and jumped to his feet. Once back in the examining room, he underwent a routine examination from the nurse. Then we were left to wait on our own for the oncologist. I can't remember what we talked about in our last few moments of hope. Because that's what we were living in: a bubble of hope about to pop. Then Randy's curiosity got the better of him, and he started searching through his medical records, which the nurse had left open on the computer.

Maybe it was better that he discovered the scan and saw the tumors growing inside him than hearing it first from the doctor.

Maybe it gave him the opportunity to see for himself, to know—really know—that the cancer cells had outsmarted all our treatments and were rapidly multiplying. We both knew that when pancreatic cancer metastasizes, there is little hope that further treatments will arrest its growth. When he blurted out, "My goose is cooked, Jai," and he started counting the tumors, Randy had accepted the trajectory his life had now taken. A cure would be next to impossible—that ship had sailed and with it our hope. His mind had embraced what his eyes saw. I, on the other hand, scrambled out of the chair to look over his shoulder. I tried to find the error in the data. "It's an older scan, not the one from this trip," I reasoned.

He corrected me. "No, it's the most recent scan. Look at the date." He started looking through more files on the computer to confirm what he believed. I told him I needed to go to the bathroom, and I slipped out the door to find the nurse in charge of the protocol regimen. I explained to her that Randy had been poking around in his electronic files and asked her to see him quickly because Randy believed he was going to die. I thought she would set him straight. He wasn't an expert on their computer system, I reasoned. He couldn't be trusted to read this information and interpret it correctly. I was searching for an explanation, not wanting to accept what we had seen: dark spots all over Randy's liver and spleen. Surely there had to be some mistake. I kept thinking this as I splashed my face and washed my hands. I returned to the examining room expecting the nurse to have disabused Randy of his silly notion.

Instead of the scene I had expected, Randy and the nurse sat there looking sad. Moments later, the oncologist entered the room and carefully confirmed that Randy had read his scans correctly: the cancer was back. He said it was as aggressive a return as he had ever seen: nine tumors in the liver and too many in the spleen to count. Three to six months of good health was all we could expect. Then he started talking about palliative care strategy with Randy.

My mind was racing to understand the turn of events. I was confused about what palliative care meant, and the doctor explained that they would now focus on slowing down the cancer in order to buy Randy as much time as possible, but the goal was no longer to eradicate the disease. I couldn't fathom the idea that my husband wasn't going to win, that he would one day very soon not be tubing with me at a water park or winning an extra-large stuffed animal. How Randy was able to accept the situation, his death, so calmly and quickly is something I'll never fully understand. Maybe he was able to disconnect his intellect from his emotions more easily than most. Maybe it was because he was an excellent chess player, former captain of his high school chess team, always two steps ahead of the game. He did his research, knew the statistical probabilities for various disease advances and scenarios, and understood that a recurrence almost always ended in death. Science was his faith, and he understood the world in which we live according to its laws. The steps for dealing with pancreatic cancer were quite clear. The first rule was to remove the cancer via surgery. The second was to kill the millions of tiny defective, replicating cells with toxic chemotherapy and radiation. The third was to get your affairs in order if the cancer comes back. In Randy's case, he had been successful in following the first rule, but had failed to succeed at the second, which resulted in the third situation. It was black and white to him.

But not for me.

"What about a liver transplant, even a pig's liver?" I asked. Randy and the oncologist shook their heads. No surgeon would do a transplant after cancer has metastasized, because by then the body's circulatory system is flooded with cancerous cells. For a successful transplant, the patient's immune system has to be suppressed, during which time the cancer would gain a foothold in other organs or perhaps in the transplanted organ. In the end, it would be a waste of resources and time. And time was precious.

I think it was about then that I started to cry uncontrollably. "That's it?" I asked incredulously, beginning to sob in one of those really embarrassing, she's-lost-it kind of ways. The doctor came and sat next to me, holding my hand. It was the first time he had ever had any physical contact with me. He usually sat in front of the computer after having examined Randy and consulted the lab results displayed on the screen. The conversation stayed in the technical realm. Now, our oncologist showed how truly great he was: he showed us his compassionate side, comforting me by talking to me in a calm and soothing voice and explaining what medical science now had to offer Randy. Randy stood watching us, an observer of the scene. I was the emotional wreck, not my husband, when it was he who was going to die. I sat there crushed, sobbing and sniffling. Cancer had blindsided me again.

When we left the examining area and entered the waiting room, I had my emotions under control, but my face couldn't hide the bad news we'd just received. Randy and I leaned on each other, holding hands as we walked past our comrades in the cancer wars.

A week after we had left Houston with our hearts and spirits broken, I was in Virginia looking at houses with my brother. It was mid-August 2007. We were putting Plan B into effect immediately, even though I had great trepidation about moving and leaving behind our good friends and strong community ties. Before I left on a return flight home at the end of the day, I put an offer down on a house. Negotiations broke off, and I went to look at more houses.

Within twenty-four hours, I came home with a house under contract and Dylan enrolled in the local public school. Now we had less
than a month to pack up our lives and move so Dylan could start
kindergarten after Labor Day.

There were many loose ends to take care of in Pittsburgh, the
sale of our house being only one of them. Friends offered to help us
in so many ways. A very generous Carnegie Mellon alumnus bought
our house and donated it to the university, which freed both time
and money for us. Others volunteered to pack up our house the day
before the moving van arrived. The school at which we had enrolled
Dylan refunded the tuition we had already paid for the coming year.
Electricity, gas, telephone, water, garbage pickup, checking, and
savings accounts all had to be terminated or closed. In the chaos,
with so many details to take care of, Randy and I were diverted
from what the move signified: Randy was going to die.

At this time, the children thought we were moving to Virginia
to be closer to my family. We didn't tell them the cancer had returned, because Dr. Reiss had advised against it, saying that until
Randy *looked* sick, we shouldn't say anything. Children have a different sense of time than adults. Dylan, Logan, and Chloe could
conceptualize today, tonight, and tomorrow. If we told them how
long Randy was expected to live, they would think he was going
to die today, tonight, or tomorrow. It's kind of like when the first
of December comes along and for the next twenty-four days, the
children ask, "Is it Christmas yet?" We didn't want to worry them
or place undue stress on them. So we acted as though our move was
a wonderful decision to live closer to family.

I kept a running list of to-do items so I didn't forget anything,
but sure enough, there were a few glitches. Packing day was a lo-

gistical nightmare. Fifteen people showed up at our house, grabbed boxes, tape, and marking pens, and got down to business. I ran from room to room answering questions and troubleshooting. We were getting dangerously low on boxes, and I had been calling the moving company, asking when they would be delivering more. Each time I called, I was reassured that the driver would be at my house any minute. Most of the volunteers had to leave by lunchtime to get back to work, and without them I wouldn't get the packing done before the moving van showed up the next day.

Then Dylan came down with a fever, and I had him rest in the back bedroom so he wouldn't be disturbed. Our sitter took the other two children out of the house so they wouldn't get underfoot amid all the people and activity.

While our friends and colleagues were packing up our worldly possessions, Randy went to the oncologist's office for his first round of palliative chemotherapy with gemcitabine. He called me in the midst of the packing turmoil to tell me his white blood cell count was low, meaning he was more susceptible to infection and sickness. "Should I take the chemo and drive my white blood cell count down lower or wait till we get to Virginia to take any more chemo?" he asked me. My brain felt as if it was melting under all the stress and pressure. I knew Randy would have a tough reaction to the drug. We were starting a two-day drive the next morning, and I needed him to be able to drive his car to Virginia. We also had a sick child whose illness could be a risk factor for Randy in a weakened condition. "Let's just wait till we get to Virginia," I said. I didn't share with him all that was going on at the house; his focus needed to be on slowing the cancer's growth. So I went back to the packing party and my sick child and called the moving company once more to find the missing boxes before I lost all my help and my mind. So many factors were outside my control. I kept trying to be that reed in the wind and bend with the force moving against me.

In this way we established a pattern: I took care of the details of our day-to-day lives while Randy concentrated on winning more time from death. We had spent a lovely summer interacting as a family, one in which there was a healthy father, but now we were moving into a different dynamic. I was slowly becoming the head of the household, making most of the decisions on my own, whereas before, Randy and I had been a team. Now I had to take the lead and rely on my best judgment. It was the start of a long and lonely road for us both. Soon, Randy's path would not only lead to various oncologists along the East Coast, but also take a surprising turn after he delivered his now famous last lecture at Carnegie Mellon University on September 18, 2007. So much had happened to us in one year. And yet there were more unexpected and challenging experiences that lay ahead.

8

The Magic of the Last Lecture

WHILE HE WAS still undergoing treatments to battle cancer, Randy had been invited to participate in a Carnegie Mellon lecture series called Journeys, in which faculty members are asked to look back on their lives and careers and offer what they've learned to their colleagues and students. When he accepted the invitation, none of us knew that the cancer would come back a month before his scheduled talk. Randy hadn't made much progress on his talk during the time he was undergoing treatment. As the date approached, he began to receive courteous nudges from the event planner asking him for a title and an abstract.

I remember the moment Randy came upon the idea for his talk. We were at Johns Hopkins Medical Center in August 2007, waiting to have the newly discovered liver metastases biopsied. Randy was working at his computer when he turned to me and said he knew what he wanted to talk about—childhood dreams. That be-

came the cornerstone for his talk, "Really Achieving Your Childhood Dreams." While we sat there in an overlit, antiseptic waiting
room, he typed up the abstract for his talk—four sentences:

> Almost all of us have childhood dreams; for example, be-
> ing an astronaut, or making movies or video games for a
> living. Sadly, most people don't achieve theirs, and I think
> that's a shame. I had several specific childhood dreams,
> and I've actually achieved most of them. More important,
> I have found ways . . . of helping many young people actu-
> ally *achieve* their childhood dreams.

As his idea became clearer, he explained to me that he could
see the role his childhood dreams had played in his life and the
many lessons he gained from the resulting experiences. Moreover,
he realized the powerful emotional return he got from helping his
students and others realize their own dreams. It was an amazing
fifteen-minute discussion, in which he talked to me and typed up
his thoughts, for I got to watch how his brain worked and how he
pulled these pieces together for the bones of his lecture. Directly
afterward, we were called back into the examining room, where
the doctor and pathologist confirmed that the tumors in Randy's
liver were metastatic pancreatic cancer. With that confirmation, we
knew he would die from the disease. The abstract he had just written a half hour before would literally be his last lecture.

Carnegie Mellon University did not bill Randy's talk in its Journeys lecture series as his last lecture nor promote the fact that he
had terminal cancer. But everybody knew because of the blog Randy
kept about his health status and because he was a popular professor.
The university community had been interested and caring about

his condition from the start. That interest hadn't waned; rather, it had increased over the twelve months he had been battling the disease. The university organizer had reserved the main auditorium for Randy's lecture in anticipation of a large crowd. Not only did the university advertise the lecture on campus, but it also contacted Randy's former students, colleagues at other universities, and collaborators from industry. Still, Randy didn't think there would be enough bodies to fill all 450 seats. Without our knowing it, word of mouth carried the news about Randy's lecture far and wide. The university also worked with Brown University and the University of North Carolina–Chapel Hill, to have the lecture streamed over the Internet to their computer science departments.

While the university was preparing for Randy's lecture, Randy and I were moving our family from Pittsburgh to Chesapeake, Virginia, to be closer to my family. Randy would help unpack the house for a while, then go work on his talk on his computer. He scanned tons of photographs and made slide after slide for his PowerPoint presentation. Randy would use a picture or some bulleted points on a slide when he gave a talk. He never wrote out exactly what he would say, but rather he would look at each slide and continue his talk smoothly as if it were written out in his head. Standing in front of hundreds of people, he never lost his poise or his place in the talk. As he composed it, I became a sounding board, listening to him try out a variety of stories told in a multitude of ways. One story in particular stands out to me. He told me about a difficult academic administrator with whom he had butted heads. He was going to use the man's real name. I suggested he call the man Dean Wormer, after the villainous academic dean in the movie *Animal House*, as a comic alternative. Randy liked my suggestion and used it in his talk. I was curious to see how all his stories would come together in the final lecture; I had only heard the talk in fragments, not from beginning to end.

By the time Randy was preparing to leave Virginia for Pittsburgh, he had amassed over three hundred slides. In addition, he had carefully thought out stage props, like stuffed animals, costumes, and his Imagineering shirt, for maximum effect. He was a master speaker who had a magical way of connecting with his audience. Randy was constantly moving slides around and deleting slides, so that the talk was always a work in progress. Deep down inside, I really wanted to hear the finished product, but our recent move and disheveled house were screaming at me. I knew he would do a great job, but I had been to a couple of these lectures before; usually there would be a small group of the speaker's friends, his students, and maybe some other professors who would attend. I wasn't anticipating that his lecture would be that different.

It was hard for me to justify leaving the children after we had moved just a few weeks earlier. For the past ten days, I had unpacked most of the boxes and figured out where to put things and how to organize our new home, while Randy scanned photograph after photograph to illustrate the points in his presentation. We were looking for a preschool for Logan, having missed the enrollment period and finding it difficult to locate a program with an available space. Chloe was still too young for preschool, which meant I needed to find child care for her so I could continue to assist Randy in a meaningful way. In addition, our house was in chaos, reflecting my own chaotic state of mind, and was enormously distracting. Boxes were piled up in the dining room and garage.

Friends and family came to help us unpack. Randy's sister Ruby and her husband, Brian, postponed their move to China and instead came to Virginia to help with the children and opening boxes. While we all settled in, Randy continued to pursue palliative chemotherapy. We found a local oncologist, Michael Lee, who was willing to collaborate with us and our oncologist in Houston.

At the same time, I began the process of looking for a nanny to help me care for the children. Our Pittsburgh nanny and angel, Laura O'Malley, had offered to stay with us for a few weeks while we looked for someone local to help us. The children loved Laura and her dog, Floyd. She had an amazing way of getting them to behave or pick up their toys by making up games to entice them. But it was unreasonable to impose on her kindness for much longer. Finding someone to replace her seemed next to impossible, but we learned about a young woman who was looking to change careers and might be willing to help us until she figured out what she wanted to do next in her life. That woman was Rachel Paige, who turned out to be one of the kindest and gentlest people I've ever met. Our children took to her immediately and, like Laura, Rachel became a member of our family.

Even with all the help from our friends and family, I was still reeling with the sudden change of course our lives had taken. I wanted to hunker down, live these last few months with Randy while he was still feeling well, and wall off the outside world with its demands on his time and attention. I wanted us to create memories for our children to hold on to for a lifetime. Nothing else mattered, in my opinion. Nothing. But my husband didn't see the end of his life playing out like that. He wasn't willing to stay at home and die quietly. He still had more living to do.

I was faced with a difficult decision once again. I recognized this was a seminal event for Randy, regardless of how many people came to hear him or what the status of our new house was. But the tugs to get our lives organized, to get our kids into a routine and help them settle into their new surroundings, and to be together as a family were compelling arguments to stay at home. Randy and I found a compromise: he would travel up to Pittsburgh the day before the event and I would follow him on the morning of it. We would stay just one night and be on the first flight next day.

On the morning of September 18, 2007, I remember looking out the taxicab window, recognizing some of the people walking down Forbes Avenue as I went to meet Randy and his friend for lunch at his favorite restaurant, Il Valletto, which was within walking distance of the university. When I first saw him, I could immediately tell he was exhausted. He explained to me that he had stayed up all night fiddling with the slides' order, rearranging the stories and the way the lecture would unfold. I was concerned that he wouldn't have the physical energy to stand up for an hour. So immediately after lunch, we headed back to campus and borrowed an office with a couch where Randy lay down to rest before show time.

After he was comfortable, my husband shooed me away to go have coffee with some old colleagues, assuring me he would be fine and would see me in the auditorium. I'd known Randy long enough to know he wanted some time to think. He stretched his six-foot frame out on the office couch, looking drained. Shaking my head, I shut the door and thought that Randy was pushing himself to the breaking point. I asked myself why he was doing this—choosing to give so much of himself to a gathering of thirty people? We had been joking about the number of people who would attend. Cleah Schleuter, the behind-the-scenes logistical organizer, kept assuring Randy he would be speaking to a full house not only in Pittsburgh, but to several university computer science departments as well.

So my surprise was twofold when I arrived at the University Center's auditorium. First, the line to get in to see the lecture snaked down the long hallway, into the lobby, and out the door. Cleah saw me and allowed me to enter the auditorium while everyone else waited until the doors opened. As I descended the steps toward the front rows, I could see VIPs already in their seats. They included former students, some of whom had flown in from California; professors from Carnegie Mellon, the University of Virginia, Brown, and the University of North Carolina–Chapel Hill; and colleagues with whom Randy had worked, including those from the Walt Disney Company and Electronic Arts. Randy had worked for Walt Disney Imagineering Virtual Reality Studio in 1995 and with Electronic Arts in 2006. Not only was there a body in every seat, but there were others on the steps inside the hall. Randy's lecture was being broadcast on campus, and additional rooms were full as well.

My second surprise came when Randy stepped out onto the stage. He didn't look exhausted or enervated, as he had been just an hour earlier. Instead, he looked . . . normal—a regular professor getting ready to give a talk. He fiddled with props and cables and looked intently at his computer for an equipment check. But I did notice that he didn't make eye contact with the audience. He didn't say hello to friends or acknowledge my presence in the front row. I read his actions as nervousness. Maybe he felt pressured to give a magnum opus with his undergraduate mentor, Dr. Andy Van Dam, present in a full house. Maybe the reality of the moment—that this would be the last time he would stand on a stage (as far as he knew) and do the thing he loved to do—weighed on his heart. But whatever it was, he tucked it away along with any lingering doubts he might have had. Randy finished his computer check and walked off the stage until it was time to begin.

After his friend and colleague Steve Seabolt of Electronic Arts introduced Randy, my husband stepped onto the stage and the magic began. It was wonderful to see him reinvigorated, his wit sharp, with his dark, cutting humor, his little smirk, his smiles. Where did he get that energy? A couple of hours earlier, he had lain on the couch in the office looking as though he needed to sleep for a week, and yet here he was, doing push-ups! What a gift Randy gave that day, in that hour, for all of us to receive. But he gained so much in return. I was so happy for him to get to realize his dream and give the lecture. From my seat, I could watch Randy enjoy his role as lecturer and see the audience's reaction to his stories and lessons.

It caught me completely off guard when Cleah rolled out a birthday cake. Randy said one of his dreams was to make other people happy and talked about how important it was to recognize the sacrifices of other people who helped us achieve our goals. He had had to leave early on my birthday, and he wanted to publicly acknowledge the time with him that I had given up in order for him to be here on this stage. Then Randy, along with the hundreds of people in the audience, sang "Happy Birthday" to me. In that moment, my heart overflowed with emotion for the man who made my life so wonderful and shared a love that was bigger than I had ever experienced. Yet at the same time, my heart broke, knowing that I would soon lose him. "Please don't die," I said to Randy when I hugged him onstage. "All the magic will go out of my life." Because he was my magic man. Without him, I believed nothing special or fun would ever happen to me or to our children again. The audience gave Randy a standing ovation. Afterward, in the atrium, he sat receiving people who stood in line to talk to him. Then we went out to dinner with a small group of people composed of Randy's research team, former students and colleagues.

For now, the magic wasn't going to stop, but rather turn surreal. A video of the lecture was posted on YouTube and became an Internet sensation. Soon Randy began receiving calls from major television network producers inviting him to appear on talk and news shows. ·

One morning in late September, Logan and I were leaving a local preschool that we had been checking out when my cell phone rang. It was Randy, excited that he had just been invited to appear on *Good Morning America* with Diane Sawyer! He began going through the logistics of flying the family up to New York City so we could all go to the studio together. Immediately, my mind began tripping over the details: What would the children wear on national television? Were they in need of haircuts? Where would the children and I be while Randy was on the set? Randy didn't care about the first two issues and explained I would have to corral the kids on a television set with cameras and power cords everywhere while he sat in a comfortable chair and talked with Diane Sawyer. *Harrumph!* This scenario was starting to have disaster written all over it. I could imagine myself trying to keep three little children quiet so their father wouldn't be distracted while he spoke on live television. I had recently wrangled the children while we took formal family portraits outdoors; that experience had left me breathless and at the end of my rope with them. I surely did not want a repeat situation with television cameras aimed at us! So I encouraged Randy to fly to New York City without us and give the interview while we watched him at home on television.

The appearance on *Good Morning America* was the first of several incredible experiences that resulted from Randy's lecture. For many of them, I chose to remain at home with our children, keeping up with the daily demands of domestic life and child rearing. Meanwhile, Randy met Oprah Winfrey and Dr. Oz, gave a lecture on time management at the University of Virginia, and spent a few hours meeting and playing football with the Pittsburgh Steelers, courtesy of ABC News and Diane Sawyer. I was thrilled that he had these extraordinary opportunities and that his final lecture had resonated so strongly with people. But at the same time, I wanted more of his energies to be directed toward our children.

Work and home life had always been an ongoing, contentious balance for Randy and me. When we dated, I could call Randy up any night of the week at midnight, and he'd still be in the lab. After we were married and had children, Randy would come home for dinner and stay until after the kids were asleep, then head back into the lab or work on his computer until midnight. The excitement and interest generated by his lecture became the new, all-consuming time sink, as his students and research had been before he became ill. I coveted every minute we had with Randy, and I loathed the new demands placed on his time, especially those that took him away from our house and our children. Randy and I were constantly negotiating the balance between his external distractions and our family.

As with other issues we faced in our marriage, Randy and I talked honestly and openly about what we were feeling. I continued to want all of my husband's time to be devoted to our family. Randy wanted to ride the wave of interest in his lecture, to allow more people to hear and to benefit from his talk, as well as to enjoy new, exciting experiences. I had to accept that it was his life that was coming to an end and that he had to finish it the way he wanted. So I had to figure out a way to be supportive of Randy and accompany him on the trips or participate in the things that he deemed important, while maintaining a normal routine and life for our children.

In the fall of 2007, our children still did not know that Randy's cancer had returned after his surgery and treatments and that it had spread to different parts of his body. They didn't know Randy's time was so limited. I wanted to lead a life that to them seemed normal in every way, so they wouldn't know by our actions that something was wrong. For example, we were not going to eat steak and lobster every night for dinner as if it was Randy's last meal. We weren't going to travel to all the places he had never visited. Many times, I felt guilty about not telling the children the truth about their father's condition, but then I would remember that they didn't have the ability to handle the stress of the knowledge that their father would die very soon. I was juggling two different sets of needs: Randy's desire to live life to the fullest before the cancer took away all his energy and the children's high demand for parental interaction.

How does one balance homework, housekeeping, soccer games, and birthday parties with talking to reporters, meeting with photographers, appearing on national television, and acting in a Hollywood movie? This didn't seem like a normal lifestyle to me, and it wasn't one to which we were accustomed. I didn't know how to explain it to our children when we had a photographer and crew come to our house at six a.m. to set up for a shoot or when a videographer from a major network shadowed us at Disney World to document our experiences and memories of the trip. Instead of trying to justify or explain the camera crew's presence, I simply presented the information as a fact and didn't offer an elaborate explanation. Because the children were so young, they didn't question me. If they did ask, I replied that Daddy had written a book that a lot of people liked. That was answer enough, and the children moved on to other interests. Randy wasn't concerned with how the children interpreted these events. His focus was on squeezing every joyous moment he could out of the time he had left. And he wanted me to share them with him.

I learned to evaluate each opportunity Randy was given and decide whether or not it was essential that I go with him. He had told me several times that he wanted me to see the Magic Castle, a Los Angeles club. Only magicians are members; they go there to practice their tricks and moves and perform shows for other magicians and guests in attendance. In the fall of 2007, Randy and I went to the Magic Castle with two friends and had the time of our lives, and Randy was thrilled that I enjoyed it as much as he thought I would.

During that same trip to the West Coast, Randy got to live another dream come true. Hollywood director J. J. Abrams contacted him to come out to Los Angeles, put on a *Star Trek* uniform, and step into the role as ensign on a Star Fleet vessel. One of his childhood heroes had been Captain Kirk on the 1960s television show. Though he wouldn't play the captain, being on the ship's bridge playing a Star Fleet officer was close enough to put Randy over the moon. He got to spend twelve hours on the set, or rather, in *Star Trek* world, meeting J. J. Abrams, talking with him, having lunch with the crew, and riding a golf cart to and from his trailer. It was an amazing experience. While Randy was sitting at his ship's console on the set, I wandered the backstage area to learn what the different people did to make a movie. I was amazed how many times they had to shoot the same scene over and over, until at the end of twelve hours, they finally were happy with the thirty-second sequence. I met the costume makers and saw where they cut out the patterns and created the uniforms. I watched makeup artists and hair stylists in action when Randy got his hair cut and had sideburns added to his new hairdo. On the set, the sound man let me listen through his headphones while the actors were speaking. I sat with the crew while the director reviewed the various takes and made decisions for the next take. But mostly I sat in a chair tucked out of the way and knitted a sweater. By the end of the day, Randy and I both had a new appreciation for directors, actors, and the myriad people who work such long hours and put so much energy into making a movie. It was also wonderful to watch Randy have a dream come true and forget about what challenges tomorrow would bring. He loved every moment of that experience, letting not a second go by without savoring and appreciating it.

In the midst of interviews regarding his lecture and once-in-a-lifetime opportunities like being an extra on a Hollywood film, Randy was approached by a Carnegie Mellon alumnus, a journalist who was in the auditorium for his lecture. His name was Jeffrey Zaslow. Jeff encouraged Randy to use his lecture as a springboard and write a book about the lessons he had learned throughout his life. I had encouraged Randy to do the same thing, calling it The Manual and suggesting he use the couple hundred slides he didn't use in his lecture. Randy was a wonderful speaker and a gifted storyteller, but he hated writing, and the idea of writing a book by himself was not appealing. With Jeff as his coauthor responsible for the text, however, Randy agreed to tackle the project. Jeff and Randy divided the work according to their strengths: Randy talked; Jeff wrote. It was the perfect partnership, and Randy enjoyed speaking with Jeff. For about an hour each day, Jeff would ask Randy questions and write down his answers and stories. Each story in the book was a life lesson Randy wanted to pass on to our children, knowing he wouldn't be there when they would be old enough to understand. The book was published in April 2008. Randy, Jeff, and I were amazed that the book became a bestselling phenomenon. The book sales, along with our financial prudence, would mean that I wouldn't have to worry about money while grieving and raising three little children. That in itself was a huge, unforeseen gift. Like his lecture that went viral and was viewed millions of times on YouTube, Randy's book seemed to strike a chord with people around the country and the world. The buzz from the lecture begat media interest at the national level, from *Good Morning America* and *The Oprah Winfrey Show*, for example. It hit the number-one position on the *New York Times* bestseller list. "Dying professor writes book on living" was how it was sensationally described. I've often been asked why *The Last Lecture* resounded with people. I think it has to do with Randy's honesty and positive outlook on life. His stories show the reader how our actions and treatment of other people have a powerful impact on the shape of our lives. That's a very empowering message and one that I'm looking forward to sharing with our children when they are old enough.

Although the media attention and cool exciting adventures added to the stress at home, Randy and I were able to strengthen our relationship and deepen our love by taking an interest in what was important to each of us and to our family. That helped us through the more difficult times to come. Still, I had to find the balance that worked for me. I didn't want death to overshadow and influence every move we made, though I wasn't trying to ignore Randy's condition, either. I think Randy worked really hard to make sure he spent time with our children, but he didn't allocate his time exactly as I had wished. I would have preferred that he be there with them 24/7.

Randy tried to minimize the impact the media had on our family. He publicly requested that people not talk about his cancer when the children were present or talk to reporters about it. He wanted to make memories for our children, like going to Disney World and having the videographer document the experience as a gift for his children later on. Soon, all too soon, Randy wouldn't have the energy to go on any adventures. His cancer would step in and demand its due. So far, we had relied upon oncologists to steer our path in the cancer war. Now we would meet another incredible advocate: our hospice nurse.

9

Unique Challenges
Caregivers Face

W E TRAVELED TO NEW YORK CITY the last week of February 2008, researching the next potential treatment to beat back those relentless pancreatic cancer cells that had outsmarted the chemotherapy drugs, gemcitabine, Tarceva, Erbitux, and Avastin. That's what makes cancer so difficult to defeat: those genetically mutated cells not only keep reproducing themselves, but they also evolve to survive in a hostile environment as the body's immune system and chemotherapies try to kill them off. With each new generation of cancer cells, the patient and doctor have to look for another treatment to attack them at a different area of weakness. Even while Randy was undergoing one therapy, we would be investigating the next potential treatment in an effort to be one step ahead. We also had to keep in mind that Randy's body was getting weaker because of the cancer's effects as well as the toxicity of the chemo, which kills not only the bad cells, but the healthy ones. It wasn't enough for the drug to be effective killing pancreatic cancer cells; it had to have tolerable side effects so that Randy could still enjoy an acceptable quality of life.

We consulted several oncologists (our local oncologist, the oncologist we worked with in Houston, and the oncology surgeon we met in Pittsburgh who cut out the original tumor) and weighed their different suggestions for therapy, looking at pros and cons. Dr. Michael Lee of Virginia Oncology Associates, Dr. Bob Woolf of MD Anderson Center, and Dr. Herbert Zeh of the University of Pittsburgh Medical Center were incredibly generous in sharing their time and expertise with us. Once we even met with Dr. Zeh on a Sunday so he could review Randy's latest lab results and give us his opinion about how to proceed next. Neither Dr. Zeh nor Dr. Woolf ever billed us for their time.

Dr. Woolf introduced us to Dr. Daniel Von Hoff, a highly regarded pancreatic cancer oncologist located in Arizona at the Translational Genomics Research Institute (TGen). Dr. Von Hoff recommended that Randy send tumor tissue samples to his research facility; there his scientists would sequence Randy's cancer cells' genome to learn which cancer drugs approved for use would most likely have a strong effect. Thanks to TGen's work, we learned that Randy's body didn't make the SPARC enzyme and would therefore be unable to process Abraxane, which in use with gemcitabine has been very successful in extending people's lives.* This information, while disappointing, was very important because it identified a drug

---

* "Abraxane in Combination with Gemcitabine Increases Survival in First-Line Treatment of Advanced Pancreatic Cancer in Phase I/II Study," *Medical News Today*, April 20, 2010, www.medicalnewstoday.com/articles/185903.php.

that would not be effective in Randy's treatment and saved us time, money, and heartache. If Randy had taken Abraxane, he would have tried the drug for three months before diagnostic imaging would have showed that it wasn't working to stop the cancer's growth. We (or rather our insurance company) would have paid thousands of dollars for the treatments. And most important, the cancer would have had significant time to grow and spread unchecked. Now we could move on to other treatments with a higher likelihood of arresting the cancer. We had very few shots left at prolonging Randy's life, and we didn't want to waste a single one. Now, based on some feedback from our doctors, we were off to talk with a couple of New York oncologists who offered unique and promising treatments for pancreatic cancer. After meeting with the first one, who confidently asserted that his treatment would buy Randy another fifteen months to live, I felt numb. *That's it?!* I remember thinking to myself. *My husband will be here next to me for only a little over a year! I'll be a widow by the time I'm forty-two!* I felt the walls closing in on me, my world getting smaller and smaller. I shared my feelings of disappointment with Randy. I told him I was scared, but I felt selfish for crying over the impact his death would have on me. He was the one dying, after all, and I wanted to be sensitive to his feelings. Randy, for his part, seemed to absorb the data in an unemotional way. He gathered the facts and filed them away to be discussed in depth with our trusted group of advisors.

The trip wasn't all doctors' visits though. It wouldn't have been an outing with Randy if some magic hadn't happened. While we were there, Randy and I sat down and talked with Diane Sawyer for an upcoming special about Randy and the widespread impact of his lecture and newly published book. It was the first time I'd spoken on camera or met a television personality. Ms. Sawyer was so personable and her staff so kind that I didn't feel nervous at all, but rather as though I was having lunch with someone I had recently met and was getting to know better. When she asked me about Randy, I felt as if I was talking with one of my girlfriends about our husbands and our home lives. The illusion would be broken by the cameraman needing to fix a light, the sound man adjusting the microphone, or the makeup artist taking the shine off my forehead. But these interruptions to our conversations were no more disruptive than a waiter coming over to take our order, refill our iced tea, or bring the bill. After the interview was over, Ms. Sawyer walked downstairs with us, said good-bye, and walked off down the street toward home as if we were friends parting after sharing a meal. It was a very special experience.

Later that night in the hotel room, I was awakened by a loud, strange noise. Looking around in the dark, I concentrated to sharpen my senses and shake the fog out of my head. What was that noise? Then I pinpointed it—the loud rasping was coming from Randy. I knew that sound too well; my first husband had been asthmatic, and I had heard him wheeze many times. Randy was wheezing in his sleep. After I observed him for a while, I went back to sleep because the wheezing wasn't severe enough to wake him up. The next morning, I talked with Randy about his labored breathing during the night, but he shrugged it off, not taking it too seriously. So I pushed my concern aside as we quickly packed up to catch our flight back home.

When we arrived at LaGuardia airport, Randy was starting to feel fatigued. With his hands on his hips, he walked lethargically and grimaced in pain. To make matters worse, our flight was delayed for several hours. Randy seemed to be fading fast, and I talked with the airline representative to switch us to another flight so I could get

Randy home. There was one seat left on a flight leaving within the hour, so Randy got on and I stayed behind. I called a friend to pick him up at the airport and prepped her about Randy's condition: lack of energy and difficulty breathing. When I got home later that night, Randy was resting, but not comfortably. His friend and Carnegie Mellon colleague, Jessica Hodgins, was visiting with us that weekend, and we tried to figure out what was going on. Jessica and Randy went to the oncologist the next morning for his weekly visit, but the nurse didn't find anything wrong, just that he had gained ten pounds in a week. This was good news, or so we thought. Randy had been steadily losing weight as a result of the disease's progress, the way it appropriated the caloric energy Randy consumed, and the chemotherapy treatments that suppressed his appetite.

That night after we went to sleep, I woke up because Randy's breathing sounded like a freight train. I was seriously scared he was going to die in bed next to me! The next morning, I argued that there must be something wrong and that Randy needed to seek medical attention. But Randy and Jessica pointed out that if there had been anything wrong, the oncological nurse would have found it at the previous day's exam. Jessica tried to act as the intermediary between Randy's position and mine. We agreed that if the symptoms continued through the weekend, Randy would call our local oncologist on Monday.

All day Saturday, Randy was uncomfortable and lethargic. He didn't get much rest that night because he couldn't lie flat in bed. He couldn't sleep on his back, and we didn't have a reclining chair for him to find a comfortable position. We tried propping him up with pillows, to no avail. Sunday morning I argued, cajoled, and begged him to call Dr. Lee, our local oncologist, but now he pushed back even more strongly, saying it was Sunday and he didn't want to bother the doctor on the weekend in the event this turned out to be nothing. He argued that in the future, when he really did need help, Dr. Lee would be less likely to believe him and come to his aid.

In my gut, I knew something was seriously wrong with Randy. It didn't seem right that he couldn't lie flat on the bed and breathe, or that he had no energy. It was killing me to watch him in so much discomfort, unable to sleep or rest, but I wanted to be respectful of Randy's choice of when he wanted to seek medical care and when not to. I called Dr. Reiss to ask her advice, and she helped us devise a compromise: Randy would call the oncology office to talk with the doctor on call and follow up on Monday if the symptoms persisted. Randy was very angry with me, saying he did not want me to hijack his health care. He wanted to be in charge of when he called the doctor and what treatments he would accept. He absolutely did not want me to act on his behalf or go behind his back. He wanted me to help him, but there was a definite line in the sand I was not to cross. I agreed to respect Randy's right to seek treatment when he felt it was necessary. But I felt it terribly unfair that I had to watch him suffer and not be allowed to do anything that could make it better. I resented that Randy did not weigh my opinion more heavily and that he was so resistant to calling the doctor to tell him about his symptoms. There would be many times when Randy would assert that he was in the driver's seat, and I was expected to come along but never to touch the wheel. He wanted me to be a part of his health care team, to go with him to all his appointments, to sit with him through the treatments, to give up time with our children, and to research treatments. And yet I was not to overstep my bounds of being "the help." I had the responsibility of caring for him without the authority to act, and it was a very frustrating place to be.

Luckily, I had Dr. Reiss and Jessica, as well as others, to talk to and commiserate with. I also used my journal as a way to blow off steam. On those blank pages, I could write anything I felt, regardless of how inappropriate or irrational it was, without hurting anyone or suffering any consequences. So often when I felt angry or scared or overwhelmed, I found that by writing in my journal I could get those feelings out—purge myself in a way. My entry on Wednesday, February 6, 2008, is pretty typical:

> Randy was up all night battling chemo side effects. I found him downstairs with his teeth chattering, body shaking, and running a 102 degree temperature. That was at 6:45 a.m. So I was running between him and the kids. I hate that. Rachel took Chloe and Logan out of the house while I got Dylan to school. Dylan was a big help this morning: he made a card for his dad, helped me paint swatches on Chloe's wall . . . Randy asked me to take his pee to the oncologist's office and pick up his Creon [a drug that helps improve the digestion of food] prescription. I ran and did that and got home in time to get Dylan from the bus stop. . . . Dinner was chaotic as usual. When Rachel left, I felt scared. Scared I wouldn't be able to take care of Randy and the kids. Randy and I got to spend time talking. He said today was what it was going to be like when the chemo stopped working. I told him this day was scary because I felt blindsided *again* by something unforeseen— where we had focused on the next treatment, here we are with renal failure. But we should learn something soon.

Some journal entries were much longer, more toxic in language than the example above, but it was good for me to get these emotions out and on the page. If the way I was feeling was too embarrassing to share with others, my journal provided a safe haven—a nonjudgmental, neutral retreat for me to escape to and express my feelings.

During this latest crisis, Randy relented and called his oncology practice. The oncologist on duty prescribed a diuretic medication to get rid of the fluid in his lungs and edema in his legs and belly. Randy's weight gain, as noted by the nurse the previous Friday, had all been fluid buildup. The diuretic worked, but not well enough. He could sleep lying down, but any physical exertion, including going up or down the stairs, left him breathless. Finally, he called the oncologist's office at the beginning of the week, and we went in for some tests. The nurse confirmed that Randy was suffering from congestive heart and renal failure. While the nurse and Randy continued discussing his condition and options, I used my Kindle to do a quick Internet search: renal failure meant Randy's kidneys couldn't rid his blood of impurities and concentrate urine, while congestive heart failure meant his heart wasn't pumping enough blood throughout his body. Once I had an understanding of Randy's condition, I turned my attention back to the conversation. Randy and the nurse talked about his appointment with the nephrologist (kidney doctor) at the end of the week. As he was leaving, I lagged behind and asked the nurse if Randy was going to die from congestive heart failure and renal failure. I wanted to know if we were at the end of our journey. I was so scared, unsure how to evaluate and respond to the information we had. Our oncology nurse told me very gently that Randy wasn't going to die right now from renal and congestive heart failure and that he would recover from these conditions. That's all I needed to know at the moment. My husband and I went home and processed in our own way what we had learned;

keeping our hopes pinned on the appointment with the nephrologist on Thursday, March 6.

On Wednesday, March 5, Randy blogged about how he was feeling during this time and what was going on with his body:

> The good news is that the tumors appear to still be basi-
> cally held in check.
>
> The bad news is that the side effects of the chemo drugs
> have become too toxic. My kidneys are now performing
> at well under 50 percent efficiency (creatinine is 3.4, and
> BUN [blood urea nitrogen] is 54, for those of you scoring
> the game at home). My blood pressure has soared up to
> 200 over 100. I may technically have "high output conges-
> tive heart failure," but that's not nearly as bad as it sounds.
>
> The painful part is that we think my abdominal cavity
> has started to fill with fluid, a side effect of the kidney in-
> efficiency and high blood pressure. That particularly stinks
> because the fluid pushes on lungs and heart. I can't sleep
> (or breathe clearly) while lying down; I have to sit up and
> try to sleep that way. And I get totally out of breath after a
> flight of stairs.
>
> So we're doing a bunch of things to address these
> issues:
>
> — We're stopping all chemo.
>
> — I'm now on high blood pressure medication.
>
> — I'm taking a diuretic that is supposed to get my
>   body to empty itself of fluids, so that my body (in
>   theory) starts to absorb back the fluid in my cavity
>   and starts to urinate it out over time.

– I'm seeing a nephrologist (kidney specialist) tomorrow.

–Yesterday I got a blood transfusion, which greatly
helped my low red blood cell count and is giving
me more energy.

This is a setback, but hopefully a small one. However, if
the damage the chemo drugs did to my kidneys is permanent, that would be really, really bad.

Randy had been keeping a blog about his fight against the disease
since he was able to type on his laptop after the surgery to remove
the original tumor. Friends, colleagues, and many of his current and
former students wanted to know how he was doing. Randy wanted
to share, but he was careful to control the way he described his situation, never getting morose or becoming emotional. As in this post
regarding his renal and congestive heart failure, he remained positive and upbeat. Sometimes I became irritated that he presented
this front on his website, keeping the darker side for me and close
friends and family to see. I interpreted his actions as an attempt
to spare people the gory details or to avoid pulling at their heart-
strings. Randy was also not expressing his own feelings about the
fear or pain he was experiencing. Blogging wasn't going to be the
place for him to vent those emotions.

After undergoing a stress test at Norfolk General Hospital to
measure how his heart was working, Randy slowly walked with me
across the street to the building where the nephrologist had his office. The distance couldn't have been more than a thousand feet, but
even that short distance was too much for Randy. He had to stop
a couple of times along the way to rest. Each time we stopped, I

offered to get him a wheelchair, which he refused. Inside the office building, Randy sat down to catch his breath. His breathing echoed loudly in the lobby, and people stared at us. I was so glad we were there to see the doctor! I just kept thinking to myself that Randy was going to get help. I encouraged him (and myself) to hang in there. Finally, he was able to stand and walk into the elevator, and we rode up to hear what the nephrologist had to say.

Dr. Thomas Whelan had an easy way about him and treated Randy as an intelligent human being with whom he could discuss the details of his condition. Dr. Whelan realized that Randy was suffering. He explained that the damage to Randy's kidneys and heart was significant enough to warrant a stay at the hospital. With the help of both Dr. Whelan and a cardiologist, Randy would have the best and safest method of recovery. A huge weight was taken off my shoulders: I was so relieved when Randy agreed to check into the hospital and allow Dr. Whelan and a cardiologist to treat him. Randy's other option had been to return home and have me administer diuretics and other prescribed medications and report back to the nephrologist and cardiologist on Randy's status. I felt totally unqualified to take on that responsibility. I didn't want to be in a position where I might miss a symptom or misread data and cause more damage to Randy's already fragile system.

With Randy's decision made, Dr. Whelan insisted on getting a wheelchair for him and pushing him from the office building over to the hospital admitting area to ensure that there were no hiccups in getting Randy admitted. Now, I've been to many hospitals and cancer centers, met a lot of caring physicians and nurses, but I have never seen another doctor have such concern for his patient as to push his wheelchair and then deal directly with the hospital administration! Not only were Dr. Whelan's actions an indication of how serious Randy's condition was, but they also illustrated what good hands we were now in. I breathed a sigh of relief, knowing it was going to be all right for now.

The Thursday afternoon Randy was admitted to the hospital, I had to scramble to make child-care arrangements, for I hadn't anticipated being gone past five p.m. Rachel, our nanny, was kind enough to stay late with the children until I could get home that night. I remained by Randy's side while the nurses set up various lines for monitors and IVs. Diuretics began to flow into Randy's body to begin the process of flushing the extra fluid out. When things seemed settled and Randy comfortable, I left the hospital to go home. Not long after the children were asleep in bed, my brother came over to stay in the house while I took Randy an over-night bag with his contact lens case and toiletries he needed. I didn't stay long. Randy was tired and would have a busy next day, and I was feeling worn out from all the excitement.

I say excitement, but really it was fear that I felt. I was so scared Randy was going to die in the hospital even though the doctors had assured me he wasn't in immediate danger. Congestive heart failure and renal failure sounded fatal, and seeing Randy connected to IVs and monitors only added to my sense that he was in trouble. I couldn't judge how much danger he was in or if he was going to die soon from these complications. I had enough experience with the children's illnesses to know when to be worried and when not to. When I got home, I was so exhausted I fell right to sleep. I didn't have the energy to even cry.

The next morning, I had to answer the children's questions about where Daddy was and when he was coming home. I told them Daddy had to go away on a business trip but would be home in a couple of days. Since Randy had traveled frequently for work, they were accustomed to his being away and didn't question me further. They had not noticed his discomfort because Randy stayed in his room most of the time. When one of the children did come into the room to see him, it was carefully choreographed so Randy had time to sit up and put on his positive, happy face. Daddy was sleeping in. He wasn't feeling too well this morning. These answers were enough; the children didn't ask any additional questions. After our nanny, Rachel, arrived and domestic tranquility was restored, I went to the hospital to be with Randy. I repeated this routine each day, spending mornings and evenings with the children and the bulk of the day with Randy at the hospital.

During the next several days, Randy's stress test indicated that his heart was working way below normal capacity. Dr. Whelan called in an excellent cardiologist, Dr. Herre, to help get his heart and blood pressure under control. More tests were done. An X-ray showed that a liter of fluid had built up in Randy's right lung, so a very long needle was inserted through his back and into his lung to drain it. Randy said this was really painful, but he felt a million times better afterward, being able to take deep breaths again and rest more easily. Randy stayed in the hospital from Thursday through Monday, until the doctors were able to get his system back on track. He had to get out by Monday, he said, so he could go to Washington, D.C., and advocate for greater awareness and funding for pancreatic cancer research in front of the United States Congress. This was just like Randy—his attention focused on something greater than himself.

Our counselor, Dr. Reiss, came in for the weekend, giving me a much-needed opportunity to discuss my fears and feelings. Dr. Reiss listened to me and reassured me that we were not at the end of the journey for Randy but that this time at the hospital was a major intersection where his health had taken a downturn.

I depended on Randy's medical team, which had grown to include the nephrologist, cardiologist, several oncologists, our counselor, and of course, the nurses who worked with the specialists. Even though I would vent my frustrations and concerns to my close friends and family, I looked to these health care professionals and their boundless experience to guide me through the turbulent waters, which became even more threatening as Randy's health declined. His body now would no longer rebound to his previous level of good health but would instead deteriorate. I confess I didn't really know when his health was taking a temporary dip or when it had moved to a new low. So I would turn to our medical team to help me understand and prepare myself psychologically to accept and deal with the consequences of his illness. Fortunately, my friends seemed always happy to listen to me, but they didn't have the skills to help me deal with the new reality each day brought.

When Randy was discharged from the hospital, I stepped up my activities in caring for his medical needs. I had to watch for weight gain and test his legs by pressing my fingers on the skin to see if my touch left a mark, indicating fluid buildup, which would signal kidney issues. I had to take his blood pressure daily and report to the cardiologist if there were any negative changes. Randy was now on eighteen different medications, some on a regular schedule, some as needed, all of which I organized in a huge pillbox a family friend had provided. I had to keep on top of his prescription refills, drug side effects, and how he was feeling overall. I arranged his visits to various specialists and made sure he got to his appointments. I took notes and followed up on the doctors' orders. Randy's health continued to spiral slowly downward. Each day and each week presented new issues, until it got to the point where I felt I needed more help to help Randy.

We needed more help at home, specifically medical help, someone who would come to the house and check in on Randy—someone who knew what they were doing! But he didn't want a stranger helping him. He didn't want someone he didn't know or trust to take care of him. He wanted only me. Randy argued that I could do it all and that I needed more child-care help. I countered that we needed a home health care nurse. We compromised. I found additional babysitting help in the event we had another emergency medical situation or our nanny was sick. Randy asked our oncologist about a home health care nurse.

That's when Wanda Wyatt entered our lives, taking the heavy burden of medical care off my shoulders, working with Randy to make his daily quality of life better, and holding both our hands as we walked that slow and scary path into the valley of the shadows. Wanda was not just a home health care nurse; she was also a hospice nurse. She started off doing simple things for Randy, like blood pressure checks, blood draws, checking for swelling and fluid retention, general performance evaluations, and dealing with medication side effects that left Randy depressed, constipated, or asleep. As Randy and I interacted with Wanda, our trust grew. From the beginning, Wanda told us she was a straight shooter and would give us her unvarnished opinion when we asked for it. Randy immediately liked Wanda; she was bright and caring. He liked that she didn't try to foist major changes on him and that her tweaks to medications really helped him. As the disease progressed and Randy's body grew weaker and weaker, we went to the oncology office less and less. In June 2008, when Randy stopped pursuing chemotherapy treatments because he was too sick to handle any more drugs, Wanda was the only medical personnel we saw on a regular basis. She came by once a week, every week, to do his checkups and offer support and advice.

Wanda became my comrade in arms—the person who could see what was really happening behind the cheerful facade Randy often wore with acquaintances, doctors, and strangers. The daily grind of cancer, pain, and fatigue takes its toll on both patient and caregiver. Wanda was able to help both Randy and me deal with the rapid changes in his condition and the chronic elements of the disease, including pain, loss of energy, loss of concentration, irritability, depression, decreased appetite, and weight loss. She knew what I was going through, not only from her extensive experience, but also from working directly with Randy at home, where his guard was down. She understood the challenges of caring for Randy, and she helped me find solutions or at least coping strategies.

I hated watching Randy in pain. It tore my heart. The cancer ravaged his body until he seemed to be nothing more than skin on bones. It was agonizing to stand by and not be able to do anything to relieve his suffering. I tried what I could: I bought a recliner chair for him to rest in. I put together a medicine chart and organized his pillbox. I would rub his shoulders, feet, or back to help ease his pain. I would sit with him and talk with him when he felt like it or sit quietly with him while he slept. It was one thing to deal with his physical deterioration, but it was another altogether to deal with the psychological and cognitive impairments.

One of the most trying issues I faced at this point was Randy's loss of memory and powers of reasoning. Randy was the smartest man I'd ever met, rational and clear-thinking. He was devoted to his children and did everything in his power to love and protect them.

That's why it made no sense to me whatsoever that he was so cavalier about the way he later took his medications. After we moved to Virginia, one of the side effects of the palliative chemo drugs was neuropathy in Randy's fingers. Without the ability to feel the tips of his fingers, holding pills was very difficult. Many times Randy would drop the medications on the floor and lose them, which was a big issue because we had little children in the house who could easily put them in their mouths thinking they were candy. I did not know what effect heart and kidney medications might have on a thirty-pound child, and I honestly didn't want to find out. With Wanda's support, I suggested to Randy that he let me put his pills in a paper cup so he could more easily get them into his mouth and would be less likely to spill them. Randy stubbornly would not agree to this plan; nor was he willing to come up with an alternate solution to what I saw as a clearly dangerous situation. It was unlike him to be irrational or to put his children at risk. But what could I do? I could have taken away all the medicine bottles and dispensed his pills as if he were in a hospital. However, this would have gotten Randy's hackles up, and there would have been no living with him. He wanted to feel in control of his life at a time when he was losing control of his body and mind. I didn't want to add to his feelings of powerlessness, but I had to protect our children.

Wanda agreed that it was a very difficult situation for my family to be in. Just her acknowledgment that I was in a terrible predicament gave me a sense of relief, a sense that I wasn't crazy or overreacting. Given that Randy wouldn't accept his medication in a cup, I became hypervigilant about checking his medicine table, his pillbox, the bedside table, the bedroom floor, the bathroom sink and floor, and the kitchen table and floor for any medicine he might have dropped or bottles he might have left open. I knew the times he was supposed to take medication, and I followed up to make sure he had remembered to do so. After checking with him, I would surreptitiously scan the areas to make sure nothing had been dropped. I had to accept that I couldn't force Randy to do things my way, but I had to keep our children as safe as possible while ensuring that Randy was in fact taking the medication he so desperately needed.

There were bumps along that road. Once, when I came in to see how Randy was doing, to make sure he was OK and had taken his medications on time, I found the pillbox empty and pills all over the floor. I was very upset because the bedroom door had been wide open and the children could have easily come into the room. When I asked Randy what had happened, he shrugged it off and said he didn't really know. I just stood there with my mouth open surveying the mess all over the table and floor: eighteen different medications, some taken several times throughout the day, mixed up and spread around. I was baffled by his nonchalant attitude and puzzled as to how this incident could have occurred. Did he fall while holding the pillbox? Not likely, I thought, because I had not heard a crash, he clearly wasn't hurt, and the medicines wouldn't have spilled out with their little plastic doors closed. Randy wouldn't have opened all twenty-eight of them. Could he really not remember what had happened, or was he hiding something? Was his short-term memory being affected by the cancer or by the drugs? What was I supposed to do to keep the children safe and still allow Randy to be in charge of his medications?

I didn't have the answer to those questions right away, so I sat down on the carpet and started picking up all the pills to refill Randy's medicine box. I could call and talk to Wanda, who would not only listen and sympathize with me, but would also talk with Randy as a neutral third party and figure out if he needed more help or had developed some new condition because of the disease. As a caregiver, one has to be hyperaware of the subtle changes in a loved one's behavior and physical aspect. Sometimes the changes are slow and imperceptible; sometimes they are dramatic, as disease takes not only the body, but the mind as well, and the pain can drive a person into a state of aggression or fear. You have to adjust your routines, your tactics, and your mind-set to keep up with ever-changing needs. The dynamics between two people who are forced into new roles as caregiver and patient can make the challenges to help, to accept help, and to love that much greater. With Wanda by my side, I had help to address these demands, and I didn't feel alone because Wanda was such a big presence in our lives.

Many times Wanda would reassure me that Randy was all right and death wasn't knocking on the door. That is, up until the second week of July when she came over to check Randy before we went up to Pittsburgh for a cancer tissue biopsy and leukapheresis, to create a customized vaccine. Leukapheresis is a process in which blood is withdrawn through an IV, transported into a machine that extracts some of the white blood cells, and is then returned through a second IV. It's a loud and scary looking piece of machinery, but the process isn't painful. At least that's what Randy said. I was terribly uncomfortable about it nonetheless. Dr. Zeh explained that once he had Randy's white blood cells, his lab would extract the dendritic cells, which are part of the immune system, mature them, and mix them with his tumor to be given as a vaccine.

Up to this point, Randy continued to pursue treatments with toxic side effects even as he got weaker and weaker. Now his system could no longer recover. The vaccine gave him hope that he could continue to fight the cancer without the terrible side effects of chemo. It would take three weeks to make from his white blood cells and tumor samples, and Randy was determined to live long enough to get it.

When Wanda came downstairs from checking Randy, I was going over child-care instructions with our babysitter, who would stay with the kids for the two days we'd be gone. Wanda and I talked briefly; she didn't think he was up for the biopsy. Always frank, Wanda said to me, "You know he's dying, Jai."

"Of course he's dying, Wanda! I've known that for months."

Then it dawned on me. Wanda had been my GPS guiding me through the twists and turns in the road. Now she was telling me we were there. We were at the end of our journey. Wanda was concerned that if we went to Pittsburgh and Randy was admitted to the hospital to undergo these two procedures, his system would fail, and he wouldn't be discharged. Then I would be in Pittsburgh with my husband dying in the hospital and my children down in Virginia with only two days of child care in place.

Nevertheless, we went. When Randy and I took our last trip to Pittsburgh together in July 2008, we were not getting along. In front of a social worker, he said he felt I was unempathetic: doing a great job of all the things anyone could do, and a terrible job on the things only I could do. Randy was usually very supportive and complimentary of me, especially in front of other people, so his comment caught me by surprise. Even though I was hurt by Randy's words, by what I perceived to be his lack of appreciation for all I was doing, I knew he was trying to tell me he needed something more of me. I heard him, but I didn't know what else I could do.

I was already walking a tightrope trying to balance our children's needs with Randy's. I couldn't imagine what more I could do, but I knew I wouldn't give up on him.

While Randy was recovering from the biopsy at Shadyside hospital in Pittsburgh, I recounted the incident to Dr. Reiss. I felt sick and angry about what Randy had said. "What does he want from me?" I asked. "He wants you to tell him you're going to miss him when he's dead," she said. I was stunned. I had been trying to avoid saying anything like this to Randy for two reasons. One, I didn't want to make him feel bad that his death would cause us so much pain, that it would cause *me* so much pain. I thought I would be making him feel guilty knowing how the grief would hurt us for the rest of our lives. Two, if I acknowledged both to myself and to him that I would miss him, I would start missing him immediately. I was terrified of the pain, of the grief that was waiting for me right around the corner. I believed that when Randy died, the magic would go out of my life. His absence would mean the end of one of my childhood dreams: to marry a man who truly loved me and to have a family. I was trying to avoid thinking about all this until I had no choice. For the moment, I could defer the inevitable. But Dr. Reiss explained to me that it was far better for me to start the grieving process now, before Randy died, so I could in fact be more empathetic to him. It was important that he see me as vulnerable, not invincible or in any way cold or uncaring. I thought by showing Randy strength I was sparing him from the fear and pain, but I was only causing a different kind of pain: a fear that I didn't love him as much as he'd thought. If I allowed the pain of loss to seep in now, Dr. Reiss assured me, it would facilitate the grieving process after Randy died.

So I went back to my husband, the man who loved me and showed me he loved me and treated me like he loved me, and I told him I was going to miss him so much when he was gone. I cried and cried. My facade of strength broke away, melted by my tears, and the raw vulnerable me showed through. And Randy was comforted. In that moment of sadness, we held each other, knowing in our hearts that we loved each other in sickness and in health, until death do us part.

10

Decisions

EVEN THOUGH OUR SURGICAL ONCOLOGIST and our hospice nurse had told me Randy was in the final stages of dying by the end of June 2008 and even though I could see with my own eyes that his health had taken a dramatic step downward that third week in July, I still wasn't prepared when, on July 25, I woke up and found Randy dead.

Randy and I had tried to prepare for this. Some of our preparations had begun before the cancer returned and metastasized in his liver and spleen. During the summer of 2007, Randy and I had met with an estate attorney to draw up his will. I became Randy's medical proxy so I could make medical decisions in the event that he was not conscious or of sound mind to voice his wishes. It was uncomfortable for both of us to contemplate the various ways he might die and difficult for Randy to articulate which medical interventions he would accept and which he would refuse. But the upside was that I knew how to act on his behalf if and when the time came, and that gave us both peace of mind. After the documents were signed and notarized, we placed them in our filing cabinet and pushed aside a portion of the anxiety that living with cancer causes.

This preparedness was part of Randy's personality. He liked to call himself a belt-and-suspenders man. In addition to coins and a wallet, Randy also carried a travel-size toothbrush, tissues, and nail clippers in his pants pockets. His laptop bag held not only his computer and power cord, but also a spare laptop battery, various hardware and networking cables, an extra contact lens case, spare glasses, and even spare underwear. It was quite in his nature for Randy to approach death in much the same way as he fortified himself to face everyday life.

The most difficult logistical matter we addressed together was Randy's funeral plans. Originally, he wanted to donate his body to medical science. Had there been the rapid autopsy programs that some cancer research centers, such as the Translational Genomics Research Institute in Arizona, are conducting today to better understand pancreatic tumor growth and evolution, I would have agreed wholeheartedly. But because that was not the case at the time, I asked Randy to allow me to bury his body, to give us the opportunity to grieve at his passing, and to create a special place for us to visit. My husband heard me out patiently, and then he agreed. I wanted to have a funeral service for Randy, as other family members of mine had had while I was growing up. I knew the ritual, its rhythm, and what to expect. Oddly enough, a funeral offered me a comfortable, familial experience, and I wanted comfort more than anything else at this time. I asked Randy to allow me to have a traditional funeral service for him, with a casket, chapel, hearse, and graveside burial service.

On Monday, May 12, we went together to a local funeral home

and worked out as many of the details as we could. That night I
wrote in my journal, "It wasn't so bad, but it made me think a lot
about how I'd like to grieve, what would make me feel comfortable.
So I was glad to get the information." With Randy sitting beside me,
it felt more like a business meeting; the ugly event itself seemed far
off in the future. Randy wasn't upset or sad during the visit. His
death didn't seem real at this point. So we were both able to keep
our emotions in check.

Like any modern office, the funeral home conference room had
a laptop projector and Internet connection to show us various casket companies' products. Our funeral home director was young
and handsome, in the prime of his life and dressed very profession-
ally. He didn't look grim or speak in whispered tones. Randy and I
each felt very comfortable sitting at the conference table with a cup
of hot tea and coffee, looking at caskets on the projection screen
and asking myriad questions. Like cars, coffins come in all sorts of
makes and models, from utilitarian to luxury. Randy leaned more
to the utilitarian ones and even considered some of the Orthodox
Jewish caskets, plain wooden boxes. Always the out-of-the-box
thinker, so to speak, Randy went one step further and explored the
option of making his own pine box. He thought he could create a
unique experience for himself by hammering together his own coffin. Very interesting idea, I thought, but I didn't think I could handle
watching Randy nail together a casket at our house! So I vetoed that
creative idea.

During our hour-long meeting, I envisioned myself at the funeral service, imagining the look of each coffin Randy considered
and how it made me feel. Later that night, I wrote in my journal,
"I'd like to go back and make the choices myself so I don't have to
contend with Randy and defer to his wishes. I'm going to be the

one sitting in front of that box, and I want it to look comfortable for him." Reading now what I wrote that night, I realize how unfeeling I sounded. It wasn't a lack of feeling, but rather the recognition that I would be the person experiencing the funeral, not Randy. The choices we made now would affect me, not him. I came to realize that the funeral is not for the dead, but rather for the people left behind, to help them give voice to their sadness and commiserate with others who feel the same way, missing someone dear and beloved. For Randy's part, it might have been a therapeutic hour in which he came to terms with his death. As always, he chose to make the best of it. However, I would be living the moment of his funeral. I would be reacting not only to the coffin, but also to the music, the flowers, the service, and the graveside ceremony. All those aspects, which for my husband were intellectual exercises or decisions to be made but not real parts of his future, would become a reality for me. I wanted it to be the softest blow possible. With Randy's blessing, I went back to the funeral home and chose a casket that looked somewhat aesthetically pleasing to me—not too ritzy, not too austere—with a satin lining and comfy pillow. These details gave me the sense that he would be at ease, even though I intellectually knew this was silly. My choices didn't have to be logical; I just didn't want them to make the moment of intense sadness and grief any worse.

With coffin selection out of the way, we turned our attention to the service. Randy wanted to keep the event small and private. He went so far as to insist that only close family be invited. We discussed the service with our minister. Later on, we had a session with Dr. Reiss, our cancer counselor, about whether or not the children should attend. Randy argued that I should not be saddled with the responsibility of looking after our children during a time when I needed to take care of myself. It isn't uncommon in other cultures for young children to attend funerals, even though they might not understand the significance of the event, but our culture tends to frown on children's attendance. We finally agreed to allow Dylan, who was six at the time of Randy's death, to make his own choice about coming to the funeral service or joining his younger siblings with the babysitter in the playroom at the funeral home. That was our compromise: I could have the children close by me on the day of Randy's funeral, but they would be in a separate area, unaware that their father's dead body lay in a coffin in the room across the hall. I made the arrangements with the funeral home in advance to set up a private room for that purpose.

When it came time to choose a cemetery plot, Randy bowed out, saying he didn't feel up to it; it had been raining for the past couple of days, and he had been experiencing pain and fatigue. I had spent the nights rubbing his feet and back to make him feel better. So on Tuesday, May 13, I went to the cemetery by myself. I called my friend, Cleah, to tell her what I was doing. We spoke for a few minutes while I walked around looking at the cremation plots, which seemed so cramped, one grave marker on top of another. I chose a sunny spot because Randy loved sunshine. No shade trees for him! I also wanted a plot away from the main road so it would be peaceful. And finally, there happened to be a playground abutting the field next to the cemetery. I liked the idea of children playing nearby, their voices carrying on the wind, because Randy would miss seeing his children grow up. An absolutely irrational thought, I know, but the detail seemed fitting and made the location meaning-ful and special to me. These three elements created a sense of peace inside me. If I had waited to pick out the burial plot after Randy had passed, I could never have thought about all these little details because I would have been an emotional wreck, overwhelmed, with family and children needing my attention. Randy didn't ask to see the plot after I had picked it out and paid for it. No doubt it was too difficult for him to stand in front of his body's final resting place.

He and I had talked at length about his end-of-life treatments with Wanda. He signed a do-not-resuscitate (DNR) order; he did not want any drastic lifesaving measures. We posted the order on the back of the bedroom door in case he had a heart attack and paramedics were called. It was helpful that Wanda had experience in this area; she led the discussion and kept us on track. Fortunately, we never had to use the DNR order, but it gave both Randy and me peace of mind. Our attorney also prepared an advance medical directive, which specified other treatments Randy wanted to have withheld from him. He declined a respirator and artificially administered nutrition and hydration, so that life would not be prolonged and he would be allowed to die at death's pace. Another document, an appointment of agent to make health care decisions, described similar wishes. It named me as Randy's health care proxy so I could enforce my husband's wishes in the event he was unable to do so himself. He also granted me durable general power of attorney so I would be able to take care of legal, tax, business, and medical decisions if he was incapacitated. We had worked on these documents from the summer of 2007 until April 2008. So much thought and discussion went into each that I felt I would truly know Randy's wishes if I had to act on his behalf.

Another topic Randy brought up during our discussions about dying is one that many terminally ill people talk about with their doctors, nurses, and loved ones: euthanasia. Randy introduced the topic by saying he did not want to linger long, an end that he felt would be a burden to me and frightening for his children. He didn't want to take up unnecessary resources, either. In his mind, the end-of-life scenario would entail his slipping into a coma for a period of time, because that's what happens in the majority of pancreatic cancer cases. If that were to come to pass, he asked me if I would give him a large dose of pain medication that would speed up the dying process and allow him to die quickly. I was stunned.

Since the time of our conversation, I've come to understand that this is a common discussion for which caregivers should prepare themselves, but I wasn't prepared for Randy's request, and I instantly recoiled. I'd given in to a lot of his requests, acquiesced to many of his wishes, but I knew in my heart I could not do this, even if I knew he would never wake up. I told him how much I loved him and respected him, but I just couldn't agree to administer an overdose. The biggest reason was that I couldn't risk our hospice nurse or some other medical personnel discovering that Randy had died by my hand. I couldn't risk going to jail, couldn't think of what would become of my children with their father dead and their mother imprisoned. Randy didn't get angry at me. He didn't try to bully or badger me, because he understood. The conversation was over, and he never brought it up again. Having asked the question, Randy knew where I stood on the issue, and I understood his fears. I would do everything I could for him—up to a point.

I know this is a sensitive topic to bring up, but it's a natural part of the dying process. I'm not advocating a particular position in regard to euthanasia, but rather trying to bring light to the fact that when faced with dying, many people will talk about their fears and possible ways to avoid living their worst nightmares, even to the point of considering euthanasia. I want to point out that the caregiver's role in health care decisions and other end-of-life care decisions is a normal, necessary part of the process. No one should be afraid to engage in these discussions or feel them inappropriate.

Even though I found our conversations difficult, awkward, and painful at the time, they benefited me tremendously. If we had never discussed Randy's last wishes or not had the legal paperwork in place, I could have been in a terrible position. I felt prepared for the worst, and I understood Randy's fears, which in turn helped me be supportive of him. With all the funeral arrangements out of the way, I could allow myself to grieve. There would have been too many emotions and too little analytical presence of mind to make well-thought-out choices. So even though it was awkward at moments, our openness to carry out the most morbid of tasks turned out to be a blessing for me. Our pragmatic approach also worked brilliantly in terms of preparing our children for their father's death.

11

———— ∞ ————

Talking to Children
About Cancer and Death

I MIGHT NOT HAVE BEEN PREPARED for the precise day and hour that Randy passed, but I felt confident in speaking with our children about their father's cancer and his death. Randy and I had spent many hours with our counselor learning about our young children's developmental stages, how they understood time and death, when to tell them about his illness, and ultimately how to break the news to Dylan, Logan, and Chloe when their father had died. To make sure I didn't forget anything, I wrote down talking points on index cards and rehearsed them over and over again. I didn't want to miss a single detail when the time came to break the sad news. I knew my emotions could easily get the better of me. Like any parents, we wanted to spare our children any pain we could, but we also wanted to address their fears and concerns so they wouldn't harbor any guilt, either.

upset the others. If I got sad or weepy, I would acknowledge that I was sad but would explain that I wouldn't always feel sad and that they wouldn't either. Most important, I wanted my children to know that they could talk about the feelings they were experiencing over the loss of their father, that I was there to take care of them emotionally as well as physically. Helping them to grieve, as well as allowing myself to grieve, became its own journey.

12

Grieving

ON THAT GLORIOUSLY SUNNY, hot summer day of July 28, 2008, I stepped into the black car reserved for the immediate family of the dead. I think it was only the second time I'd been in a limousine. I rode with my mother-in-law and Randy's sister while the sitter drove my children separately so they could return for lunch and naps. As our close family and friends began to arrive at the funeral chapel to celebrate Randy's life, I stripped off my managerial persona and gave myself permission to experience Randy's funeral service. Everything was in place. All the details were taken care of, and my children were fine. There was nothing demanding my attention. I didn't have to keep it together for anybody, to show my strong side so as not to scare my children or sadden my husband. I wasn't going to stop those sad feelings from bubbling up. I wasn't going to distract myself from the pain of the moment. Randy had been right: the funeral was my time, my opportunity to set aside all the responsibilities of home life and turn my attention to myself.

I entered the chapel after almost everybody was seated. I walked up the aisle accompanied by my sister-in-law and best friend and took the very first pew. Directly behind me was Randy's immediate family: his mother, his sister, and her family. To my left were Randy's pallbearers, including my two brothers, Bob and Rick. The rest of the chapel was occupied by our friends, Randy's graduate school buddies, and my family members. Randy's oncologist and the co-author of the book, Jeffrey Zaslow, also attended, but as Randy requested, I kept the funeral private. And that was a good thing because it made the service much more personal and intimate. Here in the safety of friends, the sadness didn't feel as heavy as when I was alone. Perhaps that was because each of us held a little piece of grief's mantle.

After the minister had conducted the service and Randy's sister had given the eulogy, people were invited to come up and share a special remembrance of Randy. Most of these stories I had heard or been witness to, but I felt comforted in hearing them again and reminiscing alongside my friends and family. And then off my thoughts would sail, floating on a story shared by one of Randy's friends about his unique and imaginative spirit. One of his longtime friends recounted some of their silly graduate school pranks. During the eighties, when Randy was a grad student at Carnegie Mellon and sharing a house in Pittsburgh with several other computer science students, he had made a birthday cake for one of the friends using granulated sugar for the frosting. Needless to say, it was rather crunchy. His friend returned the favor by making a birthday cake out of Jell-O and frosting it like a real cake. The story led me to

think about Randy's amazing baking skills. He could make check-
erboard cakes and had even made wedding cakes. He whipped up a
cake shaped like a blue crab for his father's eightieth birthday party.
The only time he shopped at Williams-Sonoma was to buy a sand-
castle-shaped Bundt cake pan.

Together we listened to some of the music Randy loved, like
"Linus and Lucy" by Vince Guaraldi. I can't hear that song without
remembering the many times Randy asked his niece to play it for
him on the piano. She always obliged, playing from memory. There
was also a slide show made up of pictures I put together showing
Randy at different stages of his life. It had been an incredibly painful project for me prior to Randy's death. But now my efforts paid
off. People laughed, smiled, and sniffled as the pictures scrolled by.

During the hour in the funeral chapel, I felt a sense of déjà vu.
There were odd parallels between Randy's funeral and our wedding eight years earlier. The same minister who married us now
conducted his funeral service. We listened to "The Rose," the song
Randy and I had chosen for our wedding, which took me back to
the sweet spring day when Randy and I held hands as we listened to
his sister sing it.

Randy and I had chosen "The Rose" because of the hope that love
kindles. Now I sat there looking at the red roses covering his coffin.
When the pallbearers lifted Randy's casket, I dutifully followed behind alone. It wasn't until that moment that it truly hit me: Randy
was dead; I was alone. I would now be walking without him beside
me. I don't know how I was able to see through my tears to make it
that short distance out of the chapel.

This train of thought led to self-pity. At the graveside service,
I reflected how instead of pronouncing us man and wife, Reverend
Herndon had committed Randy's body to the earth, releasing me

from my wedding vows "till death do us part." The crazy thoughts that run through one's mind at these moments! I admit I secretly patted myself on the back for having fulfilled my marriage vows in my second marriage. Given that my first marriage ended in divorce, I had wondered about my ability to make a marriage work. One of the silver linings of caring for Randy when he was ill was that I learned a lot about myself, including the fact that I could be a good partner, that I could work through the tough times and not be just a fair weather wife. But I had not been ready to relinquish my role as wife to the most caring and loving man I had ever met—the man who truly was my better half. Through knowing him and learning from him, Randy had made me a better person, though we had our disputes. What would become of me now that my better half was gone? What did that leave of me? The lesser half? The worse half? I honestly can't recall what the minister said at the graveside service. My thoughts dragged me down a rabbit hole from which I could not escape.

When I planned Randy's funeral, I had wanted to end it with a meaningful gesture, so instead of our minister sending everyone on their way at the conclusion of the graveside service, he invited people to come take a red rose and lay it on Randy's coffin. I had the honor of beginning. Taking the rose in my hand, I thought about our wedding song, "The Rose." Making my way to my husband's coffin, I remembered all the red roses and flower arrangements Randy had sent me when we were dating long distance and even after we were married. Standing in front of his coffin, which was poised over the open grave, I carefully laid a rose on top. I spoke to Randy. I told him I was so sorry he had died. That's when waves of grief gripped me hard. I was paralyzed—I literally couldn't move because I was shaking so hard from crying. Tears streamed down my face. I couldn't even move my hands from the coffin to wipe my eyes. I stood there overcome for what seemed like an eternity, all the while telling Randy how sorry I was. I held on to his coffin, using it as a crutch to prop myself up. Finally, my sister-in-law came up to me to ask if I was OK. "I can't move," I told her. She helped me pull my hands free from the casket and supported me while we walked to the funeral car. Once out of sight of the grave, I slowly pulled myself together. I was embarrassed by my reaction and by my display of emotion. I hadn't intended to break down like that in front of everybody, and I have no idea how people reacted to what they had witnessed. Mercifully, my family has never brought it up to this day. Sometime after the funeral, I realized how good it felt to have a good hard cry, to not be strong or have to worry about others. The funeral might have been the first time I felt such heart-wrenching emotions. It wouldn't be the last.

The funny thing about caring for someone with terminal cancer is that I had a long time to process the idea of Randy not being in my life, of Randy being dead, of being alone in the world without him, of being a single parent. When I was at the pool with just the children while Randy stayed home, I would think, "This is what it's going to be like when Randy's not here anymore," and in such moments, I would grieve for the life I was losing. When I say I was grieving, I don't mean I would break down in tears. Rather, I was conscious of how dramatically my life was going to change, and I felt remorseful, wistful, and sad. Dr. Reiss, our counselor, had told me it was good for me to allow myself these little moments of grief. That would lessen the blow later on.

For several months before Randy's death, once his cancer had spread from his liver and spleen to his lungs and peritoneal cavity, Randy began the process of shifting his attention from this life to the hereafter. He slowly lost interest in worldly events, upcoming presidential elections, for example, something he would have read about and debated vigorously. One morning, Randy told me he had seen his dead father sitting in the room with him. He wasn't upset, but rather curious about the event. I knew from the hospice literature that this was a common experience for people close to dying. We both understood that the clock was ticking away. After months of worry and fear, after living in the shadow of death and witnessing the pain of letting go of life, Randy's death came as somewhat of a relief to me. I could let go of Randy or at least the role of caring for him. I could stop trying to save my husband by running him to experimental treatments. I could quit obsessing over every change in his health status, stop worrying that even the smallest symptom, like bloating, could be a sign of something more serious, such as kidney failure. The strain of keeping him alive each day, which weighed terribly on me, was now gone.

Caregivers often feel guilty about wanting their loved ones to stay alive, while knowing that only death will bring them peace. We also learn through the media that caregivers and patients alike should appear stoic and strong in the face of pain and death. Ted Kennedy's battle with a brain tumor was a perfect example. But being worn down by the all-consuming, never-ending demands of caregiving is not a reflection of one's lack of dedication or love for a loved one dying. I suffered silently alongside Randy. I couldn't detach myself from the situation—from my job as caregiver—to recharge my batteries and come back refreshed. Caregiving is not a nine-to-five job with an hour off for lunch. My thoughts and actions revolved around Randy, whether we were physically together or not.

Luckily, I had a friend to whom I could talk about my feelings without fear of being misunderstood. Her husband was dying of cancer around the same time as Randy, and she shared with me her own struggles coping with the new, intensified battle her husband fought as he was slowly losing his grip on life. "When will the suffering end? When will God be merciful and take him home?" we asked each other as the pain and complications increased exponentially during the final several months. It wasn't that either of us wanted our husbands to die, but it was so hard to watch their slow decline as cancer advanced through their bodies, causing a loss of physical and cognitive functions. Every week there would be another health complication from either the cancer or the chemotherapy, compounding the growing list of ailments and issues Randy experienced: gut pain when he ate led to his eating less, which in turn led to fatigue, which in turn led to depression and sleeping, which suppressed his appetite even further. The cycle only intensified. There wasn't any respite from the changes in Randy's health status, leaving neither Randy nor me time to adjust to his latest condition. We tumbled together downhill until finally death released both of us from this horrendous embrace and Randy was finally at peace.

Even though I knew his death was imminent, even though I had thought about it and tried to imagine what my life would be like after Randy was no longer there, I was unprepared for the forceful blow with which grief hit me. What a misperception I had of the magnitude of the emotional response I would feel in the hours, days, and months following Randy's passing! Those little, gentle waves of grief I allowed myself to experience before his death turned into tsunamis of sadness that would roll in, crash over my head, and drag me underneath. I remember comparing the viselike grip grief had on me to labor contractions. During labor with Chloe, my body followed its natural rhythms and responses—muscles contracting, unbelievable pain that took my breath away, and exhaustion. How strange that giving birth should feel to me so similar to losing a loved one.

With my young children constantly around, I didn't want to be overcome by emotions and have them witness my intense bouts of weeping. I didn't want to scare them or upset them. So I tried to find a way to vent my feelings in a more controlled way. For example, in the weeks and months after Randy died, I would turn on the computer after the children were asleep and click on an interview with Randy just so I could see his face and listen to his voice. The first time I did this, I remember being shocked by how healthy he looked. He had been so physically ravaged by his cancer at the end. Maybe that's why Randy wouldn't let me take pictures of him at the end of his life: he didn't want me or anyone else to remember him that way. It was wonderful to push aside the final images of him being sick and instead see him as he had been during most of our lives together. But viewing those interviews came at a price. Seeing him alive and healthy tore the scabs off my tender wounds. I bled anew each night as I heard his voice and listened to him formulate responses in the way that only he could do. My heart and body ached, and tears released once again. The grief bottled up inside me needed to come out like a poison.

This was the best time for me to tackle my grief—when my children were asleep in bed and unlikely to see or hear me crying. This was also the time of day when Randy and I had shared un-interrupted moments as a couple, when we would catch up with each other, holding hands and cuddling on the couch. Now that he was gone, the silence and absence after the children were in bed screamed to me that I was alone now; the videos of Randy I watched were the perfect ingredients for creating my grieving brew. I drank long and hard from that potent elixir many nights until finally it had worked its magic. I could bear the evenings once again, and my sadness was in check.

Grief manifested itself not just in crying jags—that would have been too kind, almost manageable. It also took on a physical form. I described it to my family doctor as heartburn, as if something was lodged in my lower throat. It made my chest feel sore. I didn't think I could take deep breaths. My nerves were also frayed—I was on edge so much of the time that I was close to tears. I found myself yelling at the children. My attention to daily life waned. Before Randy's death, I was always on time in paying our bills and keeping up with domestic demands. Afterward, though, paying the bills seemed like an overwhelming task. I began to miss the little details that kept the household running smoothly. The petty issues of life caught me on their hooks, snagging me and bringing me down. And the scariest part was that I didn't want to get back up. Normally, I'm a fighter. I try to identify and solve problems. But now, I didn't care—and yet I had to, because I had three little people depending on me.

At that moment, the world seemed cold and unkind, always demanding and never giving back joy. My counselor and I had been looking for signs of depression so we could address the situation as soon as possible. I needed to be strong for myself but mostly for my children. I couldn't take a three-month hiatus to descend into darkness, to sit in a chair and retreat within myself until the wounds had healed and I could come out into the light again. I'm embarrassed to admit this, but I agreed with my counselor and my best friend that I was depressed and anxious, and I began taking antianxiety and antidepressant medication a couple of months after Randy died. The medication worked, and no longer did I have the tightness in my chest, nor would I cry at the least little thing. I didn't feel angry or overwhelmed. My children and I were happier. I was managing. Not that I didn't feel sad at times, but sadness wasn't my default mode. The dark emotions churning inside me seemed to have quieted. The medication was a short-term fix. I needed that extra help until my mind and heart healed enough for me to carry on.

I also found the support of family and friends essential when I couldn't appreciate the little joys in life—when grief seemed to cover me like a wet blanket, smothering the last rays of hope. But grief is just one of the challenges I faced as a new widow and single parent of three small children. In the upcoming year, I would find many more demons lurking in the shadows as I began to adjust to my new situation in life.

13

The Year of Firsts

L ESS THAN TWO MONTHS after Randy died, I turned forty-two. Randy had presented me with a birthday cake at his last lecture, and four hundred people sang "Happy Birthday" to me. That event is forever inextricably intertwined with my turning another year older. Under normal circumstances, that happy experience would have been an everlasting gift, but in this case—with Randy gone—I could not help but think about how magical that moment was and how I would never experience anything like that again because the man who brought the magic into our lives was gone forever. It was neither healthy nor helpful for me to reminisce about the past and dwell on what I no longer had. I had to do something to distract myself. The perfect opportunity came along in the form of a dinner invitation from my brother. To celebrate my birthday, he proposed dinner with a few friends at a fancy seafood restaurant in Virginia Beach. Dinner out might seem like a mundane event, but this little trip gave me something to look forward to, something positive I could focus on to help push aside the negative. Since Randy's death, I hadn't had anyone with whom I could go to a nice dinner or a party. Instead, I'd been anchored in my daily routine of taking care of children, other domestic responsibilities, and the never-ending paperwork that follows in the wake of a relative's death. The very process of dressing, fixing my hair, and doing my makeup was nothing short of exciting. While I was getting ready, rejecting this blouse and those shoes, I didn't think about Randy or the fact that I was a young widow. No sad thoughts wormed their way inside my head. That time was a gift in and of itself.

During the forty-minute drive to the restaurant, my brother and I caught up on each other's lives, laughing much of the time. I didn't often travel to Virginia Beach, so I looked out the window to check out the sights—the sun starting to set on the horizon, the traffic in early evening, the houses along the route, the boats for sale at the marina, and then the restaurant sitting by an inlet of Lynnhaven Bay. As we made our way across the parking lot, I wished I hadn't chosen high heels; I was obviously out of practice wearing them, and the ground was uneven. Once inside the restaurant, I found myself captivated watching the people at the bar, imagining their lives. The sunset reflecting on the water was mesmerizing. I was completely absorbed in the newness of the excursion, the fine food, beautiful view, surrounded by others and sharing the evening with friends with whom I could engage in stimulating conversation. I didn't feel sad during those couple of hours. Randy's absence wasn't paramount in my mind. Instead, I was enjoying the moment, living my life as it now was without a feeling of regret for what it once was.

So began my Year of Firsts, which is what grief counselors call the year following the loss of a loved one. This period presents special challenges to the person grieving because it demands trying to reconcile the past with the present. With each holiday and celebration, I wondered how to handle the family traditions we had established, now that Randy was no longer with us. In addition to the logistical details that had to be decided, each date would also conjure up painful memories. Anticipating an upcoming event, I tried to decide how best to take care of myself in order to minimize any stress or sadness I might experience. Maybe our holidays and rituals would follow the same routine Randy and I had established; maybe I would create a new tradition, or a blend of old and new. Even if one thing worked for the children and me during this tender year, it didn't mean we were committed to repeating it in the years to come. So I felt free to set aside the way Randy and I always used to do things and focus on what worked for us at this moment. I didn't have to be handcuffed to the past. I had to learn to give myself the freedom to do what was best for my family.

But as the fall days ticked away, I could sense a growing sadness. We were approaching our first Christmas without Randy. Actually, that's not true. We had to celebrate Christmas 2006 without him when he was undergoing chemotherapy treatment in Houston, but I had known that our family would be reunited. Now there would never be another Christmas with Randy helping to put the star on top of the tree or baking Christmas cookies or watching the children open their presents. Christmas 2008 and New Year's 2009 were particularly painful holidays. Instead of excitement, I was feeling blue, dreading even the arrival of Christmas morning and time with my family. I moved into a hyper decorating mode. I wanted to distract us with beauty. I hung pine garlands throughout the house, from our vestibule up the staircase, over every doorframe, even from the kitchen light fixture and pot rack. Poinsettias, angels, Santa Clauses, children caroling, bowls of golden pears, and shiny ornaments added to the festive mood. There was a seven-foot Christmas tree blocking the back door. The children had a wonderful time decorating it. But then came the moment when the star awaited its ascent to the top of the tree. We all looked at each other because Daddy was the one who would lift up Dylan, the oldest and most capable child, to place it there. How was the star to make it to the top now that Daddy wasn't here? We were looking directly at the loss of our family tradition—such a small but symbolic gesture, and we had to deal with it. We discussed our options. Even with the stepstool, none of the children was tall enough to reach the top of the tree. Dylan said I should put the star on top now because I was the tallest. But I had another suggestion: I offered to lift each child up so that everyone would have a turn putting the star on top and then taking it off for the next person. I would be the last to put the star on top. Everyone liked that plan the best, and a new family tradition was born. Someday the children will get to be too big and heavy for me to lift, but I'm confident we'll be able to create a new tradition when the time comes.

Christmas Day presented similar, though more complex logistical adjustments. I had already learned some tricks of handling the opening of gifts once the children woke up. After Christmas 2006, I took the toys out of their boxes, removed the plastic packaging and wire ties, put batteries in if necessary, tested the toys to make sure they worked, and then wrapped them up. That way, when the children unwrapped their gifts, I didn't have three little ones begging me to hurry up and get their toys out the packages so they could play with them. Because Santa makes his own toys, they are always ready to be played with—no assembly required, right?

My extended family offered to change holiday commitments and schedules in order to come to our house for Christmas lunch. My mother, father, uncle, aunt, and brother and his family were to bring several dishes, to make the meal preparation easier for me. I had to bake the turkey and biscuits. Of course, there was still cleaning up the house, setting the adult table with our best tablecloth, plates, utensils, and glasses, and getting the card table out of the attic for the children. I still distracted myself by trying to re-create a Currier and Ives scene, but I in fact created a more stressful situation. Dylan, Logan, and Chloe wouldn't remember how the table looked or if there was wrapping paper left on the floor from the morning's chaos. They had a very special time spending the afternoon with their family and playing with their cousins, and that, to me, made the effort worth it.

The next morning, the children and I visited Randy's family in Columbia, Maryland, to spend time with Randy's mother, Virginia, his sister Tammy, and her children, Laura, Christopher, and Micajah. Tammy's husband, Al, wasn't able to make the trip because of work commitments. The children and I were supposed to take a short flight there, but the flight was delayed for several hours, so I canceled our reservations and decided to drive the four hours instead. I had thought flying might be easier than navigating I-95 and Washington, D.C., traffic on a holiday, but with a three-hour minimum delay, I wasn't going to risk getting stuck at the airport with the children. This was my first time driving to Grandma Pausch's house by myself from Virginia, and it was the first time we had visited her in over a year. Before Randy got sick, we would go to Columbia from Pittsburgh once every couple of months! Randy always drove. My brother was worried and cautioned me not to undertake the trip by myself. It had started to rain in the late afternoon, and the winter sun was waning behind the clouds. I weighed the option of waiting a day and starting out fresh the next morning. If we didn't leave that day, we would lose out on spending time with Tammy and her family, who had to leave the following day. I asked myself if I could drive four hours while minding the kids. How would I handle bathroom breaks with three children? Was I putting my children at risk by driving them to their grandmother's house? I decided that I could make it by myself. I talked to the children, telling them I needed their cooperation, that I needed them to listen to me when we went into the bathrooms at the rest stops. I promised to call my brother when we arrived. Then, with a full tank of gas, we headed down the highway for Grandma's. I was in the driver's seat, both literally and figuratively. I had to determine what was best for my children and for me. The responsibility never felt heavier, and Randy's level-headedness was never missed more. But there was something exciting about setting my own course. I could feel a spark of my own magic beginning to flicker.

Happily, we arrived safe and sound in Columbia with no mishaps to report. There was only one jarring occurrence. I got confused as to which highway to take after bypassing Washington. The GPS was telling me to take Highway 29, but I remembered Randy taking a different route off 95 to get to Columbia. Without thinking about it, I turned to the passenger seat to ask Randy what to do. Of course, the seat was empty and my copilot was no longer there. My brain was so used to his being beside me, it had reacted automatically. *He's not here to help guide me,* I thought. *I'm on my own.* And I began to cry.

Unfortunately, there would be more trying moments at Randy's childhood home. I felt as if he was present, like a specter. Pictures of him could be found throughout the house. Randy's face, as a child, teenager, or adult, smiled at me from every room. At one point, Chloe asked me to follow her from the kitchen to come see her daddy. She took me to the living room and pointed to a picture of Randy with his family at an amusement park. "That's my daddy," she said. "Yes, it is, darling," I responded. "Wasn't he handsome?" But she didn't answer. She had already wandered away to play with her brothers, leaving me to stare into the eyes of the man I had married and with whom I had created this beautiful family.

The boys were curious about the pictures Randy painted on his bedroom walls when he was a teenager. Logan lay quietly on the bed looking around the room at the silver elevator, the submarine periscope, the footprints on the ceiling, the heart over one of the twin headboards, the message in a bottle, the quadratic equation, and the chess pieces. Dylan wondered out loud about what his father had been thinking when he painted the submarine, which then led to a discussion about their father and his high school interests. There weren't any tears during our talk, and neither boy seemed sad, just interested in the boy their father had been. What remarkable, unforeseeable consequences painting his room created! More than thirty years later, Randy's children were learning about him from those pictures.

After the children were in bed in Randy's old room, Virginia, Tammy, Laura, and I shared stories about our Thanksgiving and Christmas holidays. We talked about all the normal things families do: how the children were doing in school, their sports activities, our work and activities. It grew late, and as we were about to say good night to each other, I asked Tammy, "Did you ever think there would be a day when I would be sitting here in your parents' house talking with you, and Randy not here?" "Absolutely not," she replied. Divorce would have been more logical than death. However, with Randy's death, we walked into unfamiliar terrain. His mother and sister continued to treat me as part of the family, for which I was

and continue to be so grateful. I couldn't imagine losing Randy and
his family at the same time. It would be too great a loss to handle.
We're still trying to figure out holiday schedules and visiting dates,
but at least I know they want to be in our lives and maintain close
ties with our children.

Being with Randy's family made the world seem more stable,
more familiar to me. It was one of the few aspects of my life that
hadn't changed. Randy's room was the same. Grandma Pausch was
the same. Tammy and her family were the same. And we were all
still family—something I could depend on and hold like a candle in
the dark. For these reasons, I felt comforted spending part of the
Christmas holidays and ringing in the New Year with the Pausches.
The love and safety I felt with the Pausch clan far outweighed the
discomfort I experienced in facing those memories in Randy's
childhood home.

After Randy's sister Tammy and her family returned home to Virginia, his sister Ruby and my friend Tina joined us. The four of us
sat around Grandma Pausch's kitchen table watching Dick Clark's
New Year's Eve television special after the children were tucked in
bed. Here among family and friends, I felt supported and loved. We
had a shared connection through Randy whom I wasn't ready to let
go of even as the old year was counting down. I was a widow; Virginia had lost her son, Ruby her brother. In their presence, I wasn't
pitied, nor was I different from them, because we were all marked
by the same loss.

Once the Times Square New Year's Eve ball dropped and we
wished each other a happy New Year, I went to bed. Lying there
in the dark in a twin bed, I thought about my last New Year's with
Randy, about how we held hands. He'd been down in the dumps
that evening, upset because of Dylan's reaction during the film *Mr.*

Magorium's Wonder Emporium, which they had seen earlier. In the movie, the toy-store owner dies, and Dylan became upset, and Randy had to console him. The episode gave him a glimpse of the grief his son would soon experience, and it made him very sad. Lying there in the dark by myself, I thought about being here in his home without him and about the new year starting without him, dragging me along with it. I felt I had done a good job of taking care of the children and myself during this particularly emotion-laden holiday. My children had benefited from spending time with their relatives and being in their father's childhood home. The visual reminders of him had not upset them, but rather had given us permission to talk openly and lovingly about him. It was also an occasion for me to experience the love and support of my extended family.

I had to keep adjusting and coping as the days passed and the holidays and special occasions kept coming. Sometimes my planning to take care of myself in advance of a special occasion wasn't successful. Valentine's Day 2009 was a good example. It had been six months since Randy's death. How could I prepare for it? I couldn't give myself a box of chocolates or a bouquet of roses. Anyway, flowers always reminded me of Randy. When we dated, he filled my office with beautiful arrangements just to remind me of him and his love for me. Every Valentine's Day, he would give me a dozen long-stemmed roses, sometimes white, usually red. He even talked about arranging to send me flowers once a year after his death, but I asked him not to because I thought it would be too painful. So on this first Valentine's Day without Randy, my friends and family wanted to be supportive of me. My sister-in-law invited me to go out with some girlfriends the night before Valentine's Day as a nice diversion. I arranged to have a babysitter watch the children for me. As we were leaving the neighborhood, I thought I saw my brother's car and asked my sister-in-law if my brother was coming to our house for some reason. She said I must be mistaken, and we went on to have a nice evening without my giving the incident another thought. When I returned home later that evening, my children were waiting to surprise me with homemade Valentine's cards that Uncle Bob had secretly helped them make and a beautiful bouquet of flowers he had bought to have them give to me. It was really lovely, but in the moment, still filled to the brim with grief, all I saw was sympathy for the poor widow. My attitude persisted into Valentine's Day with the addition of several more bouquets of flowers from friends and family. Each vase represented to me an attempt to fill the void of Randy's roses. All I could think of was that I would never again receive flowers from him. He was gone, and so was our love. Sadly, in this mind-set, I couldn't see the love and support filling up my house with the arrival of every flower and card. Grief blinded me and blocked out the beauty and love being offered to me.

Later on, I thought about how I had viewed the Valentine's gifts as symbols of loss. I decided I didn't want to live my life feeling that way, shunning the love of family and friends who were trying to help buoy me up in difficult times. I had a choice of how to live my life: I could choose not to miss out on the wonders and joys that life had in store in spite of Randy's death, or I could wallow in self-pity and grief. In that moment, I chose to push back against the gray and see that not all my life was sadness. There were rays of sunshine and beauty. I just had to be willing to see them.

That was a challenge I faced with each holiday and special occasion. I learned to listen to myself about what I needed in order to get through the difficult times and the overwhelming feelings of sadness. I had to consider what worked best for our family so as to meet our needs during the Year of Firsts. I was slowly rebuilding my life, giving myself permission to dream new dreams. Even as I took these small steps, Randy wasn't forgotten. Choosing to live and finding ways to nurture and support myself didn't erase the pain or the loneliness, but the effort helped. Sometimes I had to work hard to push past the self-pity, which could engulf me, and to reframe an event to see the sweetness that is still there in my life. Slowly, without my being aware of it, I was learning how to move forward.

As the clouds of grief and fear began to dissipate, I started to think about how I wanted to live my life. I didn't feel guilty about leaving Randy behind. I didn't love him any less because I created new holiday traditions. He was a part of me, a part of the family we had made together. I learned how to manage the past without compromising the present. Most important, I was learning not to look at today through the lens of yesterday, which made the promise of tomorrow all the more magical.

14

———— ⌾⌾⌾ ————

Untethering Our House
from the Past

SOON AFTER WE WERE MARRIED, Randy and I went shopping together—a very rare event because Randy hated shopping, especially for himself. When he needed new clothes,
he'd set out like a soldier on a reconnaissance mission into enemy
territory—his objective was to get in and get out as quickly as
possible. His closet held only one style of pants: Dockers, khaki,
pleated, no cuff. His shirts were typically polo shirts embroidered
with the logo or name of some conference he had attended. I, on
the other hand, could find pleasure browsing in a store, though it
wasn't a major pastime for me. One beautiful summer day, we set
off to try out mattresses and compare prices. Randy always believed
in getting three quotes on a product or service to make sure he
had chosen the best deal, so we had to go to at least three different
stores. By the end of the day, we had successfully agreed on a firm,

pillow-top king-size mattress. Randy had really wanted the king-size because, as he said, he wanted the bed to be large enough for our future children to snuggle with us on weekend mornings or in the evening. He had fond memories of piling into bed with his parents, and he wanted to continue this tradition with our children. A few days later, our mattress arrived. And later on, as Randy predicted, our children did get into bed with us, sometimes too early for our taste, but it was a wonderful time for cuddling and talking with our little ones.

We had made so many plans together lying in that bed and dreaming about our life, our family. Our talks, our arguments, our whispered secrets to each other were woven into the very fabrics in our bedroom. With so many powerful associations, they naturally triggered thoughts and memories of Randy. I avoided the room, and even after shifting the furniture around, I still couldn't shake my uneasiness. I couldn't sleep in there, so I retreated to the guest room, passing in and out of the master bedroom to get dressed and quickly get out.

While I was trying not to evoke Randy's ghost, my oldest son, Dylan, wanted the bedroom to stay exactly the same. Dylan reacted strongly against any changes in the house. He cried when we moved the bed to a different wall not long after Randy died. He said he wanted everything left as it was so he could go in the bedroom and remember when he and his father snuggled in bed watching *MythBusters* or telling stories. By stepping into the room, Dylan could visualize Daddy when he was alive. He didn't want to lose that strong tether to the past, and I respected his wishes and feelings.

For Dylan's sake, I didn't remodel the master bedroom. I didn't relocate the television we had given Randy for his forty-seventh birthday. The entire room went unused for several months. I left everything as it had been before July 25, 2008, until I finally felt that things had calmed down, that we had a bit of a new routine established and we could feel life's forward momentum pulling us along. The past was still present with us, but eventually it became sounds in the background that we were able to tune out at will.

As my children and I learned to make peace with Randy's absence and to live with his memory, I went back into the master bedroom and took a hard look at it. My objective now was to make this space mine, to make myself comfortable in the house where I had to live. I had to make our house into my home, and it was time to redecorate. Of course I missed Randy, and of course my heart still ached. But I needed to move forward with the rest of my life, starting in the safety and intimacy of what had been our room.

When I came back up to the master bedroom, the room Randy had convalesced in and died in, where we had shared our last moments together on this earth, I felt all the sacredness of those experiences. I thought I was strong enough to handle all the emotions I would feel in this place. However, it took months to even begin the process. With Randy gone, the same bed that had seemed at times too small now felt way too big. At night, I felt swallowed by the emptiness around me, I missed my husband so. There was no one, no body to fill up his side of the bed or to wake me up getting into bed after I was already asleep. It was colder without my furry space heater, as Randy often referred to himself. Without him, the world seemed a more hostile place.

In the mornings when I was half awake, I would reach for Randy before realizing he wasn't there. My hand would find the indentation where his body used to be, created over our precious years together. Morning after morning, I would wake to the feeling of loss and the reminder of my new status as a widow. My heart would break anew. I couldn't go on this way. I couldn't wake each day to feel my loss both literally and figuratively.

I suffered needlessly in my attempt to balance my love and memories of Randy with my need for peace and tranquility. Finally I decided I would never lose those experiences we had shared together in this room, or in any other for that matter, regardless of whether I painted the walls or the house was destroyed in a hurricane. They were and are mine forever, for me to reflect on and honor at the time most appropriate for me. What I didn't want was for this space to trigger memories when I was unprepared. Unlike my children, I didn't want it to be a shrine to the past. So I began my makeover with a hopeful outlook. Soon I reveled in listening to myself, deciding what would make me feel comfortable and happy.

I started by taking care of the immediate reminder—the mattress. My friend Roger Magowitz, owner of Mattress Discounters in Virginia, had told me to call him if I ever needed a mattress, and he would help me find something that worked best for me. This would be my first step to change something so closely associated with Randy. In his thirty years in the bedding business, Roger had learned that one of the most common reasons people buy a new mattress is the death of a spouse. I guess he had foreseen my inevitable need. I accepted his invitation to answer my questions, knowing I wouldn't have to explain why I was buying a new mattress; I wouldn't have to talk about Randy's death. The past would remain there and not intrude on the present, when I could focus on the pleasure of shopping for myself.

What a treat it was lying on all of the different kinds of mattresses in the store! It was also a novel experience not to have to negotiate or compromise with someone else. It was just my opinion that mattered—such a change in the way I had been thinking and operating for many years. Between caring for babies and then Randy, my wants and needs had often gone last or unrealized. Now I was listening to myself and finding I could make changes to suit myself without feeling as if I was betraying the memory of my husband. The experience was rejuvenating—awakening in me a dormant drive to take care of myself. Just as I had learned to make new family traditions in accordance with what would work best for the children and me, I was now beginning to see I could exercise the same principle in other areas of my life.

Next I pitched out all the old bed linens: the pillows we had bought, the sheets we got at Sam's Club on sale—all gone! I started fresh. I painted the bedroom a deep shade of blueberry. I got rid of the Luxo lighting that Randy had insisted on for utilitarian reasons and I had disliked for aesthetic reasons. I bought beautiful lamps and curtains. I hung new pictures on the walls and put a chaise longue in the corner to make it feel like a retreat just for me. Down went the ceiling fan; up went a pretty light fixture. By the time I was done, the room was completely transformed. The chains to the past were broken! I had surrounded myself with beauty that made me catch my breath each time I walked into the room. More important, Randy's ghost wouldn't haunt me in here any longer.

Next I turned my attention to our bathroom, with its double sinks. Even after I removed Randy's toiletries, I could still envision him at his sink brushing his teeth and putting in his contacts, leaving toothpaste residue in the bowl and contact lens solution seemingly everywhere. The empty counter and useless double sink were a powerful visual reminder of my husband, who was no longer there to greet me in the morning with a smile and kiss in the continual dance we call marriage.

I'd always wanted a place to sit down to put on my makeup, so

I wouldn't drop my eye-shadow applicator or mascara wand in the sink. I had gotten pretty good at basic plumbing, having put in new single-lever faucets in the children's bathroom. So I decided to rip out one of the double sinks, cap off the pipes, and cut down the cabinet with the help of a neighbor. I was going to make a vanity table for myself.

I had a long to-do list, which is still not complete.

Many people who lose a loved one choose to move from the house that holds so many memories. My friend with two young children sold her house about a year after her husband died. She told me of the pain visual reminders caused her—the flooring they had put down together or the deck he had built. I was lucky that Randy and our family had moved into our house in Virginia only eleven months earlier. Our house couldn't tell the same kinds of stories. I also couldn't move because of my children. Randy and I had talked at length with our cancer counselor and to a child psychologist before we decided to move to Virginia. We wanted to know what effect moving would have on the children after Randy died. Should we move closer to family before he died or stay put in the comfort of the only home they knew? Randy felt very strongly that it was important to be closer to family so I could have a support network to help raise our children. And both professionals said it would be better for our children if we moved before Randy died. Being in the same house after he passed away would give them stability and a sense that their father knew where they were.

Many books advise grieving spouses not to make any major changes during the year following the death of their beloved. I can appreciate the idea of a year as being the yardstick to measure how long it might take to get one's emotions better in check. But I don't think it should be a hard-and-fast rule. We all grieve in individual ways, with different degrees of emotional intensity and varying needs. I found I needed to get control over the space I had inhabited so it wouldn't cause me to tear up every time I rose in the morning. My son, on the other hand, wanted memories of his father associated with various rooms throughout the house to remain. I tried to find a time frame that worked for both of us, recognizing that we were sharing the same space and missing the same person.

So I didn't always follow the "wait a year before you make major changes" rule. For example, I asked Randy's friends to help me clean out the clothes, shoes, and sporting goods from his closet while they were in Virginia for the funeral. I didn't need twelve months to give away his clothes to people who could use them. Not all of Randy's possessions went to Goodwill. A hospice volunteer took three of his shirts and cut and sewed them to fit cute little teddy bears, which she then gave to our children.

Furthermore, not all memories are bittersweet; some are just plain bitter. Like any normal couple, Randy and I had our disagreements. One issue arose over deciding on a new car to replace his thirteen-year-old Volkswagen Cabriolet. This coincided with his finishing the trial chemotherapy treatment in the spring of 2007. That was before the cancer had returned and metastasized to his liver and spleen—a time when we were hopeful he would beat the disease. I encouraged Randy to take this opportunity to buy a new car as an affirmation that he was going to live. I wanted him to drive this new car into the ground over many years, just as he had his Cabriolet. He agreed but said we should choose this car together. We had several fun outings test-driving convertibles, for Randy was a ragtop man. It gave us something else to think about besides the cancer and what might happen next. We could live in the moment, without worrying about tomorrow.

But independent of my input, Randy narrowed the field down to two cars. I no longer felt that this was a couple's decision or that I was really part of the process. When it came down to deciding, I expressed my feelings and said I felt my opinion on the final selection should carry more weight. Randy disagreed. Maybe he felt this would be the last car he might ever get to buy if his cancer returned. Maybe he thought he deserved to have the ultimate say, since he had suffered so much in fighting cancer. I don't know exactly what was going on in his mind; he rarely articulated what emotions or thoughts were driving his actions. Finally he told me I could sell the damn car after he was dead and go buy whatever I wanted. That ugly statement just hung in the air for a few minutes. I held my tongue so I wouldn't say anything I would regret. I was so disappointed in Randy, not only for the comment, but also for the way he had acted during the whole process. I ran through all the unhelpful things I wanted to say in return, but I didn't vocalize them. Instead, I told him that if the car meant that much to him, he should pick out what he wanted, and I would step aside.

Randy went on to buy his first choice, and for obvious reasons, I never did like the car. He loved driving around with the top down, enjoying the fresh air. Ironically, he wasn't able to drive or even ride in the passenger seat after the cancer had spread through his system. The car had too hard a ride. Given the damage that had been done to his organs, every bump in the road caused him pain. So the car sat in the driveway, and it was rarely used after Randy passed away.

The car became a negative reminder of our argument and the un-charitable feelings I had had. I didn't wait a full year to sell it—just a couple of months to make sure the children would be OK with Daddy's car going to a good home. Then I followed Randy's orders and went out to buy what I had always wanted—a Mini Cooper

Clubman with really good gas mileage and a backseat big enough for two children's car seats. It's bright yellow with white racing stripes and white and black flames on the side. My brother calls it a clown car, but it makes me laugh every time I see it and smile each time I drive it. I'm glad I didn't wait a year to bring a little joy into my life. And I needed a daily laugh, especially as the burden of being a single parent became greater with each passing day.

15

Single Parenting:
My New Frontier

NEAR THE END of Randy's battle, our house was a three-ring circus, and I was the reluctant ringmaster. In ring number one were the kids, whose activities were supervised by our nanny, Rachel. In ring number two was Randy with his health issues and emotional needs. Finally, in ring number three was the endless stream of visitors, from family members and friends to hospice care workers. Rarely was I ever in the house alone with Randy and the children. We had so much support, so much help to make it through the worst of times, for which I am forever grateful. But all of the activities made our household chaotic, to say the least.

Then suddenly the merry-go-round stopped spinning. The children and I felt a little dizzy, a little unbalanced in the aftermath of Randy's death. The buzz of activities we were strangely used to was now a hum instead of a roar. Visitors stopped coming to our house.

The phone didn't ring quite as often. This slowdown naturally happens after someone passes away, but it is an adjustment phase for the family left behind. Ours was no different. We were living in transition, trying to find our new normal.

Transitions are always difficult, whether you're adjusting to a death in the family, unemployment, retirement, divorce, or any other major life change. For me, the transition was multilayered. I was grappling with widowhood, grief, single parenthood with three small children, and my new unemployment as a caregiver. I know *unemployment* sounds like a strange word, but caring for Randy had been my job, my focus, and a large part of my daily routine for two years. During this time, I had a lot of help with the children. Now that role and routine were gone. What was left was a void I had to face and fill. I had to create a new routine with my children, just as I was doing on a larger scale with my life.

Though I was grieving for my husband and reeling from his absence, I never let our everyday life come to a standstill. I didn't feel I had the luxury of lying in bed, nursing my sorrow and focusing only on myself. For Dylan, Logan, and Chloe, I kept putting one foot in front of the other, balancing my needs with theirs. This feeling of responsibility for them has had nothing but an upside for me, keeping me anchored in the world of the living and able to feel their love and experience their joy. I've never lost sight of the fact that my children are one of my many blessings. Because of them, I have learned how boundless love can be. My love for them makes me want to be the best person I can be, as well as a good parent. In teaching them kindness and how to be courteous to others, I've relearned these essential lessons myself. I feel highly motivated to help them be happy and well adjusted, to give them experiences that allow them to learn about their world, and to instill in them the values Randy and I shared. I could not—and would not—let them down as their only parent in the wake of their father's death.

My children challenge me to meet my lofty parenting goals every day. As a rule, my kids wake up ready to go at six o'clock in the morning, if not earlier. They're energetic and physical, so we get moving and do a lot before most people are out of bed. The downside to their energy is that they totally wear me out, especially when I'm in the backyard playing hide-and-seek and other games with them. There isn't a second parent to tag team with when I get tired.

After a full day of activities with me, the children no longer had Randy's homecoming after work to divert their attention. They missed having him come home and take an interest in their day, talking with them and looking at their art or schoolwork. Instead, the children vie aggressively for my attention. Dylan and I were talking recently when he was home from school sick and no one else was around to interrupt us. I asked him what it was like from his perspective to have one parent raise him. As he put it, now "There's one source of energy in the family: Mom. The three power plants want the energy. We have to share. If it's not distributed equally, the power plant needing more energy would send out calls and Mommy would notice because of the fighting."

Dylan speaks just like his father—he even uses analogies like him! More to the point, he realizes that fighting with each other is a way to get my attention. Sometimes children will make bad choices to force an adult to interact with them, even if that interaction is negative. Perhaps they wanted my attention because I had been so caught up in Randy's care that they felt neglected. Perhaps they were dealing with the loss of their father and the changes in their lives by acting out with each other. Regardless of the reason, it made parenting even more difficult. One of my family members even took me aside and told me people were talking behind my back about how ill-behaved my children were. Well, that didn't make me feel very good, to say the least! I could blame myself and lose faith in myself as a parent, but I realize those folks only see my children for a fraction of the time I do. To the contrary, I've seen a huge improvement in their behavior. The trauma they went through obviously had a big impact on them, but they've readjusted and ac-climated. They've also matured as they've aged, which has helped as well.

Another big help was Rachel, who stayed with us for about six months after Randy died. This gave the children a sense of continu-ity. It also enabled me to adjust to my new situation. However, the time finally arrived, the day I had dreaded, when Rachel was ready to move on with her life. She had come to help us while she was in a period of transition herself, trying to figure out a different, more fulfilling career. We assumed we would need her help for about a year, given Randy's three-to-six-months prognosis. But when Ra-chel told me she had decided to be a teacher and was enrolling in education classes, I found myself both scared and shaken. I wasn't prepared to lose yet another person in my life, as well as the only partner I now had in raising my children. There were several issues in play here. It wasn't a question of finances. Randy had encouraged me to keep a nanny for some time after he had passed, just to make our lives more manageable since he would no longer be there to help out. We looked at our finances and budgeted for the child-care expense. The real issue for me was that someone to whom I had become close was now leaving our daily lives. I was experiencing another loss. I didn't have the heart to try to replace her because I couldn't bear to bring another person into the privacy of our home to become close to us and then leave us after a while. I didn't want to be hurt anymore by people coming and going from my life, and I definitely didn't want the children to go through a series of care-takers coming in and out of their lives. I worried about attachment issues for them. Then there was the blatant criticism I got from friends and family; the message I heard was that I was a bad mom for having child-care help.

With my decision made, I still worried how I would manage alone. When would I get a much-needed break or a little time for myself without regularly scheduled child care? I questioned how I would manage when the children got sick and needed extra at-tention and I had to function sleep-deprived for days. In the fall of 2008, for example, the children came down with hand, foot and mouth disease, the stomach flu, and a random virus that brought on high temperatures. And that was in the three months before winter set in and the cold and flu season officially started. I wasn't sure I would have the endurance and energy during those times to care for them without a partner or regularly scheduled help. Of course, I still had my family and friends to lean on in emergencies, which I did. Once I had to call my brother Bob at six o'clock in the morning after stomach flu traveled through everyone in the house and finally made its way to me. To his credit, Bob was at my house in fifteen minutes and stayed with us for most of the day, allowing me to rest and recover. But helpful friends and family were there for emergen-cies, not for me to call when I needed a nap because I had been up all night or when I wanted to go to the gym to work out. With our nanny leaving, yet another aspect of my life was in transition.

Shortly after Rachel left, I found a woman who could come ev-ery Tuesday and Thursday afternoon to watch the children for me. I also developed a long list of high school and college students whom I could call on, though I quickly learned that trying to find a high schooler who was free on a weeknight so I could attend a parent-teacher conference was a project in and of itself. Another downside was that my young children had to adjust to many different people, with different personalities and ways of doing things. And that would not bring out the best in their behavior.

Moreover, I was struggling with the extra demands that complicated everyday life. I felt like a sailor who had learned the basics of sailing and then went out on a boat and battled stormy seas. I needed calm, stable waters until I had my sea legs under me. But life doesn't wait, and I had to meet whatever challenges came my way. One of the earliest and in some ways most common challenges was juggling the children's schedule. Making sure everyone has their homework done and done correctly, plus staying on top of the extracurricular demands—special projects, field trips, and sports—takes a great deal of energy and attention. In the spring of 2008 when Randy was very ill, Dylan started playing soccer. He played the next season after Randy had passed away, but I found it too draining to try to watch him while entertaining the two little ones on the sidelines. Logan wanted to play a sport as well, but I didn't know if I could manage the usual schoolwork routine, plus two different practice and game schedules. Luckily, we found a compromise by choosing an activity both boys could enjoy: Tae Kwon Do. By now, in the spring of 2010, Chloe was three and was content to play for forty-five minutes while the boys practiced. Soon, though, the boys were at different belt levels, which meant different class schedules. We were now struggling to make the recommended three Tae Kwon Do classes a week, which was difficult and stressful for everyone. Dylan had also added violin lessons to his schedule, which were given at his school after classes were over. Once a week, Chloe and I would drive the thirty minutes to school and meet the boys. On days with good weather, they would have a snack and play on the school playground. Dylan would have his thirty-minute lesson while we remained outside. After his lesson was over, we would pile into the car and get home by five p.m. Tasked with getting the children to school in the morning, picking Chloe up by one p.m. and the boys by four, and then starting the after-school activity schedule, I felt I was constantly on the run. By Christmas 2010, I found myself losing my temper more often and feeling depressed. I struggled to keep my head above water. My brother suggested we cut out some commitments to reduce the time demands. Dylan put violin lessons on hold, and the boys went to Tae Kwon Do class only once a week. I felt so guilty that I couldn't give the children the opportunities to play sports or learn musical instruments. It made me feel like a failure as a mom.

Finally a friend pulled me aside and told me she was concerned about me. We talked about what was bothering me, and she suggested I look into getting someone to help with the children and their schedule. She suggested an au pair, who would live with us in exchange for room and board and pocket money. At first I thought getting child-care help again would be an admission that I was less of a mother. But I had these children with my husband who had committed to raising them with me. Randy once calculated that he helped me with child care about sixty hours a week. He had strongly encouraged me to keep some child care in place after he had passed in order to help fill the gap created by his absence. After Rachel left, I thought I would be able to do it all on my own, but that effort came at a high price—a price I wasn't willing to pay. I wasn't the best parent I could be—far from it. I wanted to be a better parent, and I wanted our lives to be better.

I took my friend's advice and hired an au pair. She helps me in the morning to get the children dressed, fed, and driven to school.

While they are in school, she takes a class at a local university. In the afternoon, we divide the responsibilities of picking up the children from school, helping with their homework, supervising or playing with them, getting the laundry done, and making dinner. After dinner, she goes out with her friends, does her homework, or hangs out with my family. The children have really enjoyed having her with us. They like helping her learn English and hearing about her country and its culture. I have seen a huge improvement in my energy and happiness. I don't feel worn down all the time. I smile more and am more easygoing.

I still miss having Randy here, though, to help me raise our children. Even though I now have help with the kids, I no longer have the man with whom I can talk over issues and make decisions. Randy's analytical strength was unparalleled, and I had come to lean on him for his insights. As a professional people manager, he was great at handling irksome situations. His skills were finely honed from running a research group and teaching classes where people learned how to work in teams. One of the greatest techniques he taught me was to start off a conversation needed to convey one's displeasure over a particular occurrence by acknowledging something positive the person did. I, on the other hand, am not the best people manager. I've learned how to distract little children when they try to put their fingers in light switches. For a more complex situation, like confrontation for example, I've had to work hard to develop a skill set. My natural inclination is to get emotional rather than stay rational and calm. I found myself in just this situation this past summer when I wanted the boys to participate on a local swim team. I thought that would not only improve their swimming skills, but also give them the opportunity to make new friends. It would also add some structure to those endless summer days. Dylan flat-out refused, saying he didn't want to do it and I couldn't make him. I was flabbergasted that he would challenge my authority. I was raised by a marine corps drill instructor and a hard-core disciplinarian, so the parental role model I had was not one I wanted to emulate. I didn't immediately respond to Dylan's statement on an emotional level, which is a testament to the effort I've made to think first and react later. First I tried to explain the reasons for his joining the swim team. Still Dylan resisted. I remained steadfast in my decision and took him and Logan to the pool for practice. Most of the time, Dylan got in and swam without giving me any pushback, but there were one or two mornings when the water was cold and he put up a fuss. Somehow I believe Randy would have handled this situation better than I did. Maybe that's raising him up on a pedestal, but I think he would have worked some magic, said the right words, and Dylan would have been more than happy to get in the cold water every June morning to swim.

I'm sure the children do the same thing: idolize their dad. Chloe was two years old when Randy died. She doesn't remember her father as a disciplinarian. After he passed away, when I put her in the "time-out" chair for some infraction, she would sit there and cry over and over, "I want my daddy!" She seemed to instinctively know that her daddy would protect her and rescue her from the evil woman who was holding her captive against her will. She probably also knew she was pushing my buttons, well aware that I often cried when we talked about Daddy. During those long, long 120-second time-outs, I tried very hard not to respond or react to her pleadings for Daddy to come save her. I tried not to show my hurt, and I stayed firm in making her sit there. As time has passed, the children pleaded less fervently and frequently for their father to swoop in and save them from the consequences of their actions.

There have also been times when I've encountered a situation that I simply didn't know how to handle. Without my partner to turn to, I learned to talk with other people—friends or the children's pediatrician or teachers. Turning to professionals helped me make informed decisions, and the process instilled me with confidence. At times, I still feel overwhelmed. I think that's true for many parents—we're frightened by the fact that our children's lives are in our hands; it's a weighty responsibility. Right after Randy died, just thinking about my role as the sole parent would inflame my anxiety and tighten the knot in my chest. I remember crying as I went downstairs one morning to make breakfast, thinking, *My God, I'm all alone. I'm really doing this by myself.* It wasn't that this was an isolated incident where I was alone to start the day with the kids, but the recognition that every day from here forward would be me by myself fulfilling the children's needs. At moments like that, I'd have to focus on getting through the next hour to prove to myself that I was going to be fine, that we were going to be fine. *See,* I'd say to myself, *I got through one hour; I can get through one day.* Each day would strengthen the base I stood on as a single parent, until finally my feet felt as though they were on solid ground.

Now that I've had some time to find a routine and strategies that work for us, parenting isn't nearly as difficult. We've become comfortable as a family of four instead of five. As the children have grown older and their interests in life have expanded, they don't seem to need my attention quite as much. I'm not at the point where I can read a book while they swim in the pool, but we're getting there. As the demands of parenting have relaxed, I've turned my thoughts to taking care of myself a little more. By nurturing myself, I believe I'll be a better nurturer of my children.

16

Taking Care of Me

I'M REALLY NERVOUS WALKING UP to the tennis court with a racquet in hand. Not only have I never played tennis before; I haven't played any sport since I was a kid and played ball in the backyard with my brother. Now I'm trying to figure out how to grip the racquet, swing, and connect with the ball coming at me. The tennis pro yells for me to follow through—bring the racquet up to my left ear as if I was talking on the phone. So I concentrate on talking on the phone over and over again while the summer sun beats down on me. It feels good to be in the sunshine and to be exercising. It feels good to be alive.

I got the idea to learn tennis from a magazine article I read in the oncologist's office in the spring of 2008. Tennis is an excellent way to manage stress, the article claimed. Given all we were going through as Randy continued to battle cancer, I was in dire need of stress management! The neighborhood pool we joined when we moved down to Virginia also had a few tennis courts and offered beginner lessons. The courts were ten minutes away and would take one hour out of my schedule. Surely I could manage one hour a week for myself.

I signed up for lessons and joined the class in May 2008. After that first lesson, I was a believer. There is indeed something therapeutic about watching for that fuzzy green ball, swinging the racquet, and feeling the connection of strings on the ball. In trying to anticipate where the ball would be and how to get my body and racquet positioned to return it, there was no room in my conscious mind for anything except the demands of the moment—no room for thoughts about Randy or cancer or, later on, my grief. No mundane tasks like making dinner or yard work could recapture my attention. For one hour, I could utterly escape the normal concerns of my life.

Playing tennis would become one of the best ways I took care of myself during the time Randy was dying and directly afterward. I didn't realize that what I was doing at the time was escaping; I just knew I needed to get out of the pressure cooker. I had tried other activities, like going for a walk or going to the gym, but neither was mentally consuming enough to give me a break from the everyday worries. I didn't spend those precious moments enjoying the breeze or sunshine; I couldn't keep my worries locked away. Instead I would spend the entire walk strategizing about what I was going to do when I got back home. But tennis was new enough and difficult enough for me that my brain couldn't focus on anything else.

Another unexpected benefit was the possibility of connecting and reconnecting with other people whom I discovered on the court. At the beginner clinic, I was surprised to run into an old high school friend. She introduced me to the wife of one of our high school friends. This was one of the great advantages of moving back home. But it's also the nature of tennis—it's a social sport. People play together on the court and socialize off of it.

I immediately joined a fall tennis league, which enabled me to play once a week with a group of women. As a result, I met fifteen new people, doubling my circle of acquaintances. The friendships I've forged have played an important part in helping me create a new identity for myself as Jai Pausch, not Randy's wife or Dylan's or Logan's or Chloe's mom. This is something we all need: a life outside and beyond one role, whether that role is as a webmaster or a stay-at-home mom. Without tennis, I would have had limited opportunities to meet other adults and establish meaningful relationships because I don't have a job outside the house.

In the wake of our move, there was a huge void—a major piece of my life I had to rebuild in Virginia. Tennis was a first step in that direction. Leaving Pittsburgh meant I left behind an active social life that I had built over the ten years we lived there. I had been involved at our church, where I participated in several social groups, like the parents-with-small-children group and a covenant group of four couples with children around the same age. After Dylan was born, I had joined the Pittsburgh Toy Lending Library, a nonprofit volunteer-run group that maintains a play space for children under five. Randy and I had participated in the Pittsburgh Sports League. Many of our neighbors were also of similar age and at a similar stage in child rearing; we would often have play dates and dinners together. Randy and I were blessed to count his work colleagues as friends with whom we socialized outside the workplace. There were mothers with whom I had become close through the preschool my children attended. Moreover, I had made friends through the gym, yoga, knitting, and creative writing classes I had taken. To duplicate this rich network of diverse people would take years. I had to build a new group of friends by taking advantage of the uniqueness of our new home, instead of trying to create the same life I had in Pittsburgh.

A more practical tactic I adopted in taking care of myself was finding a way to feel safe in the house at night. It's funny, because when Randy was alive, he was too sick to have protected us in the event of a burglary, but just his presence was enough to make me feel safe. After he passed away, though, bedtime became a time of high anxiety for me. As the quiet of the evening enveloped me after the children were asleep, the emptiness of my bed would awaken my sense of loss and aloneness. I would hear the house's night noises, and my active imagination would conjure up robbers or trespassers in the house. On and on as the clock ticked, my mind would torture me with one horrible possibility after another until, finally exhausted, I would fall asleep, only to be awakened shortly thereafter by a child who needed comforting. I am lucky to have family living so close by, yet I was all alone in my room at night battling those anxiety-fueled demons. I had to figure out a way to comfort myself at night, and a night-light wasn't going to do the trick.

My aunt suggested the perfect solution: a house alarm. The company installed sensors on all the doors and windows and put in a motion sensor too. When we left the house, I could set the alarm and feel secure when we returned that no one had broken in and was hiding somewhere. The house alarm helped to allay my fears when I heard a noise in the middle of the night. I knew it was nothing to worry about if the alarm hadn't gone off, so I could go back to sleep and get some rest. A side benefit was a feature that notified me with a chiming sound whenever the front or back doors were opened, even during the day when the house alarm wasn't set. If a child went outside when I was upstairs moving laundry around, I would hear the chime and investigate what was going on and could more easily keep up with the children's whereabouts. All in all, this simple decision has given me great piece of mind.

While I was rebuilding my life in Virginia and slowly creating a new life for the children, I told myself that I would do something special for myself when the children graduated from high school. This was a long-term goal—a dream I wouldn't realize for at least sixteen years, but it gave me something to look forward to. When I had a bad day, I would think about my special plan and I would day-dream about what it would be like. My dream started off simply: after the last child had graduated, I would take a trip to Paris, France, a logical choice because my undergraduate major was in French language and literature. I had traveled to that magical city three times in my life and just loved it. It was easy to reminisce about the good times I had had there and look forward to enjoying new ones after the children were grown. My dream grew in relation to the growing difficulties and challenges of each day. One week was no longer enough of a payback for sixteen years of putting off my needs to take care of others. No, it would have to be a whole year. Yes, that's what I'd do. After I gave everything I could to raise my children to the best of my abilities, I would follow one of my dreams and spend a whole year in Paris.

For a while, this trick worked really well, but then I thought about how unfair I was being to myself to put off my dreams for sixteen years. I love to travel and have been fortunate to have visited many interesting places at home and abroad. Why should I have to give up completely my passion for travel? Couldn't I find some way to take some limited trips *now*? What if I waited until the children graduated only to find out I had some health issue that prevented me from achieving my dream? How would I feel then? Bitter, no doubt, and very angry, with no one to blame for the lost opportunities but myself.

My best friend, Tina Carr, whom I've known since my days as a webmaster at Carnegie Mellon, suggested we take a trip together to Italy, focusing on just Rome and Venice to make the trip manageable and not exhausting. Wow! Just the thought of seeing the ancient Roman ruins, the Vatican, and the light in Venice made me giddy with joy and anticipation. It took me about six months to plan and prepare for the trip. The most important part was to find a sitter to stay with my children for nine days, a huge job and the linchpin of our journey. If the children weren't being well cared for and I wasn't one-hundred-percent confident in the person watching over them, I would never enjoy the trip. Luckily, I had been using a woman who had chosen professional babysitting as a second career. She was very experienced, mature, and trustworthy. As an added bonus, she had babysat for me many times, and the children knew her very well.

When Tina and I boarded our flight to Rome, I was over the moon with excitement and anticipation. We had read through our guidebooks and planned our itineraries. I had practiced some Italian phrases, but I figured I'd rely on my ability to speak French and Spanish to get by. We managed just fine. The Italians were polite as we tried to communicate in poor Italian, mingled with French, Spanish, and English. It was a refreshing change from speaking "preschool."

Of course I enjoyed the historical sites that Rome had to offer, but one of the things I enjoyed most of all was sitting at breakfast and enjoying a hot cup of coffee with warm, frothed milk on top. I didn't have to jump up from the table to fetch something or clean up a spill. Instead I sat quietly, watching the Romans walk past on their way to work while I enjoyed my steaming hot coffee.

After four days in Rome, Tina and I packed up and prepared to take the train to Venice. But instead of being excited about the next leg of our journey, I felt sad. I found myself missing Randy terribly and wished we had been able to go to Venice together as we had always said we would. The grief swelled inside me until I felt I would burst. I cried standing in a beautiful Roman hotel room because I was going to the lovely city of Venice. I felt like such an idiot. But Tina was completely understanding. She just hugged me and reassured me that those feelings would pass and I would enjoy Venice even though Randy wasn't with me.

She was partially right. Venice was beautiful, especially as the sun set and the light reflected off the water onto the buildings. It was an incredible sight to behold. Saint Mark's Cathedral was spectacular, with its medieval architecture and its astonishing history. But the first night we were there, I didn't think I could bear to remain in the city. There was so much romance everywhere I looked. Everywhere I looked I saw couples—young couples smooching, middle-aged couples still in love and holding hands, old couples having dinner together. At the outdoor cafés in the square were several orchestras playing music that encouraged couples to dance together. Love was literally in the air. There were the gondola rides—happy couples sat side by side as the gondolier paddled them through the canals and, for a little extra, sang in Italian. Seeing these twosomes, especially the older ones, drove home my loss: my husband was dead, and we would never be in Venice together to dance a waltz or enjoy the sights or, on a larger scale, grow old together. It was so depressing that I decided to return to our hotel. My heart felt bruised. To top off the evening, our hotel neighbors made loud, passionate love.

Tina had slept that first evening; she had stayed at the hotel fighting a migraine while I was out exploring the city. Refreshed and ready for a new adventure, she was shocked by my sadness and disappointment. Over my favorite hot cup of coffee with frothed milk, she helped me laugh off the previous evening and look around at the beauty surrounding us at that very moment. Just in front of us was the main canal with boats going by and the sun beaming down. My spirits lifted as I took in what I had been blind to only hours before. With Tina's help, I pushed back the veil of sadness that had been covering my eyes and saw the richness that surrounded me. I was determined not to lose this fantastic moment. Picking up my guidebook and sunglasses, I rose from the table ready to enjoy my life as it is now and to stop living in the past.

The next two days were wonderful. We walked along the pathways, taking in the sights, getting lost, and then finding our way back. We decided to take a gondola ride in the middle of the day when it wouldn't be such a romantic setting, and as we walked around we surveyed all the gondoliers until we found one who was very handsome and seemed nice. Thanks to Tina's silly disposition, I laughed so much during the ride that I never once found myself thinking about my loss. Tina also has a lovely voice, so she sang for us. Not a shrinking violet, I piped up a stirring rendition of "Row, Row, Row Your Boat," which became a duet and then fell apart as we both collapsed in laughter. The rest of the sightseeing went pretty much the same way, the two of us acting like silly schoolgirls, laughing and taking in as much of Italy as we could, making the most of every moment we had.

Since our Italian journey, I have taken a couple of other short trips—to Washington, D.C., and to the Caribbean to celebrate Tina's birthday. During each one, I recharged my batteries and returned home ready to resume my responsibilities. I feel I can give more of myself after doing something for myself. But tennis and travel aren't the only ways I have found to escape the pressures of my daily life. I've also learned to take a little break during the day or in the evening to lose myself in a book. During the flight to Italy, I had started the Twilight series by Stephenie Meyer. Now, I'm not ordinarily a paranormal or romance novel reader, but I downloaded the book after several of my friends told me they had read it and really liked it. I found myself addicted to the story, so much so that I read and reread the novels multiple times. When I had finished reading the first book, I scoured the bookstores in Rome to find the second. Then in Venice, I had to find the third. After I finished the fourth book, I started all over again. And again. When I talked to my counselor about this strange obsession, not understanding why I seemed stuck in this story, she explained that this, too, was an escape for me. Whenever I had free time, especially in the evening when I felt lonely, I could pick up a book and immerse myself in another world. The Twilight series was pure escapism, an easy read without a complex narrative full of characters and plot lines to challenge my already overtaxed brain. I couldn't handle Marguerite Duras or Virginia Woolf with their complicated storytelling techniques and sentence structures, even though I had been a literature major in college and enjoyed intellectually stimulating novels. I identified with the main characters; the pain Bella felt when she lost the love of her life and the blank pages representing her withdrawal from the world were so very similar to what I was feeling. It was a cathartic experience that made me feel better after having released some of my own emotions in a safe way. After reading for a little while, I could put the book down and return to my life, ready once again to face my world with all its joys and sorrows.

Though I feared that the magical, extraordinary events we had experienced because of Randy would disappear from our lives after he passed, I came to realize this worry was unfounded. As I took small steps to move forward with my life and create opportunities for myself, I saw that *I* could make some magic happen too. Slowly I would once again come to believe I had everything I really needed, right here inside me. I wasn't dependent on someone else for excitement or interesting activities. I had the power to create these elements by myself, for myself.

17

Magic: Lost and Found

WHEN RANDY PRESENTED ME with my birthday cake in front of four hundred people during his last lecture, I knew the moment we were sharing was probably the last amazing act of love my husband would ever show me. How many men would have the forethought to make their wives part of their last opportunity to do the thing they love most? Standing on that stage with him in front of all those people, I was feeling so happy and yet so sad at the same time. I loved Randy so much, and this was just one of the many reasons he was precious to me. And yet I knew he would be gone soon. Not only would the love of my life disappear, but also the amazing *Wow!* experiences in which he involved the kids and me. Without his spark, our lives would seem dark—or at least that's what I believed.

Randy was all about experiencing life with a sense of inquisitiveness, always with a smile on his face. He didn't care about possessions. Doing things together, spending time with each other—that's what mattered most to him and to me. We had begun raising Dylan, Logan, and Chloe to value family time and adventures. Without Randy, I didn't believe we would have any more unique trips, but I found that I simply couldn't give up on the idea of having cool experiences or time with family members who live out of town.

Water parks were always high on our list of favorite things to do. We had season passes to Pittsburgh's Sandcastle Waterpark, where we'd take the children even when they could enjoy only the baby pool and we had to take turns watching two kids while the other zoomed down a water slide. When we were dating, Randy and I had traveled as far as Orlando to experience Disney's Blizzard Beach, which Randy thought was one of the best water parks. We'd spend hours and hours in the pool, going down the slides, and floating aimlessly down the lazy river. Much to my surprise and consternation, Randy got me to do the 120-foot-high body slide, through which you descend at speeds of 50 to 60 miles per hour and drop twelve stories. Once was enough for me, but Randy did it over and over again, enjoying the thrill each time. Even with the Whipple surgery's giant scar running down his entire torso, Randy did the high-speed slide at Sandcastle, announcing triumphantly after he reached the bottom that his stitched-up body had held together. He was so full of life that he made even the simple things like a water slide seem magical.

I wanted to recapture some of the magic I so sorely missed, and I wanted my children to know how exciting life can be. During the 2009 spring break, just six months after Randy had passed away, I took the children to an indoor water park in Williamsburg, Virginia. After talking with friends who had been there with their children, I decided I should be able to keep my children safe; if we got there and I was concerned that the situation wasn't foolproof for my crew, we could drive the hour back home and try again when my kids were a little older. But I desperately wanted to have fun just as we did when Randy was alive and healthy. I missed that part of my life.

So I packed our suitcase and buckled them into car seats and booster seats and drove north to Williamsburg. After we had checked into the hotel, the kids and I were excited to get to the pool, so we quickly changed into our bathing suits. I took off my watch and earrings and put them in the hotel room safe just before we left. When we passed through the hotel area into the water park, the awe on my children's faces was priceless. I knew they had inherited the water-park gene from their father and me. Surveying the scene, we saw at least four different pools, including a kiddy pool, a wave pool, a deep pool for big kids, and a lazy river. In the middle of the pools was an imposing play structure with interactive water guns, water shoots, rope ladders, and body slides. There was even a big inner-tube slide at the far end of the area that we could all do together. Our excitement was palpable, and the children were ready to run off to play. They were like a herd of wild horses, tossing their heads and pawing the ground, ready to bolt.

I stopped them. We talked about how to be safe and reviewed the Rules, which included staying where Mommy could see them, no roughhousing, no running, and no peeing in the pool. Happily for me, there were life-preserver vests to fit Logan and Chloe; there were lifeguards in every pool and on the play structure, too. With all these safety features built in, I felt sure they weren't going to drown even though I couldn't keep my eyes on each of them every second. Chloe, who was almost three years old, wanted to stay in the baby pool with its little slide and tiny water chutes and shallow water. Logan, four and a half, and Dylan, seven and a half, wanted to be on the play structure or in the wave pool. I compromised by letting the boys cavort on the play structure while Chloe and I were in the baby pool. After a little while, we went together to the wave pool, where Chloe played on the shore and the boys enjoyed jumping in and riding on the waves. To my surprise, Chloe was allowed to ride in the tube with me and the boys. So off we went to slip down the big slide in a huge tube. I was a little nervous, so I put Chloe in my lap and Logan and Dylan on either side of me. Then down, down, down we went, twisting and turning, squeals of delight ringing loudly in the air. We got to the bottom safely with everyone laughing. Even little Chloe enjoyed it. My thoughts instantly turned to Randy and how he would have been thrilled to see how much his children loved the water park. It was a bittersweet moment for me, but I didn't allow myself to dwell too much on these thoughts. I didn't want to darken the moment, and honestly, I didn't have time to indulge my grief. I had to run after the children, who were ready for the next thrill.

After several hours of playing in the water, we were all exhausted and went back to the room for a nap. The children were hungry when they woke up, so we got ready for dinner and went out to the hotel restaurant. This is the part of vacations I like best—not having to plan or cook a meal. At some point during the dinner—I think it was when I went to pay the bill—I looked at my hand and noticed that my diamond engagement ring was not on my finger! I began to panic, searching through my purse and around the table in case it had fallen off. No such luck! The children could see how upset I was and tried to help me remember when I had seen it last. I couldn't remember when I had last looked at it because I never took it off. My stomach was doing flips, and my heart was breaking.

This was the diamond Randy had given me when he proposed marriage on one knee in my grandparents' house. On our fifth wedding anniversary, he had it reset for me in a bezel setting so I wouldn't scratch the children with a prong. That ring had never come off my finger before in all the times we had been at a pool, beach, or water park. I never gave a thought to taking it off, since it hadn't slipped off before. I had moved the ring to my right finger when I started getting eczema on my left ring finger about a month before Randy died. When my skin would flare up red and itchy, I would move my ring to the other hand until it cleared. Lately I'd been wearing it on the right hand. Maybe the right ring finger was slightly smaller. Maybe the ring fit a little more loosely because we'd spent all day in the water. Maybe the ring slipped off while I was speeding down a water slide with Chloe, Logan, and Dylan or while we were all playing in the wave pool together. Regardless of how or when it disappeared, the fact remained: my engagement ring was gone! I was completely devastated and distraught.

The four of us rushed back to the hotel room, and the children helped me search everywhere. I began to cry when it didn't turn up. I was so upset, so angry with myself for not taking the ring off and putting it in the safe with my watch. When we didn't find it in the room, we went to the front desk to inquire if someone had found it and turned it in. The desk clerk made some phone calls, but no ring had been turned in. The employee told me to go see the pool manager in case it had been trapped by one of the filters. So the children and I went back to the water park and talked with the manager, who said she would check the drains and filters that evening after the park closed. I'd have to wait until the next day to see if my ring had been found.

That night, I was angry at myself and the world. "What more could possibly happen! What more could go wrong?" I asked myself. Here was our first big adventure in which I felt we had reclaimed some joie de vivre. In my mind, I tried to reframe the lost ring in a helpful, positive way. On the one hand, my engagement ring was a physical reminder of our marriage and our life together; no other ring could replace it or represent my husband's love. After I had calmed down a little, I was able to take a more rational view of the situation. In my heart, I knew the ring was just a thing. It was a sentimental thing, but a thing nonetheless. I hadn't lost anything of *real* importance or value. This wasn't a tragedy in the true sense of the word. No one had drowned, gotten lost, or gotten hurt. Nor would I lose any of the loving memories or the loving feelings I associated with the ring. In fact, losing the ring led me to an epiphany of sorts. Here we were, having a fantastic day at the water park. The kids and I were laughing and sliding and splashing like crazy. We were having one of those wonderful experiences I had been so afraid we'd never have again. I saw that the magic hadn't gone out of our lives when Randy died. The magic was still with us, inside us. It always had been. I could lose a tangible part of Randy and a symbol of our marriage, but I could never lose the magic we created together. Was I glad I lost my ring? No! But what I had gained in going to the water park was more valuable than any material object. This trip put me one step further along on the road to rebuilding my life.

Furthermore, if I had to lose that ring, then I thought the water park was a good place for it to rest. I found peace in thinking about that ring lying at the bottom of a pool somewhere. Maybe a good man would find it and give it to the woman he loved and wanted to marry; it would be a symbol of another couple's love. I hoped in my heart that that couple would experience the kind of love Randy and I had had—a love that I would never stop feeling, with or without a ring on my finger. Even after death has parted us, I still feel it today.

Since the water park adventure, the children and I have gone on to enjoy many amazing experiences. In the spring of 2009, we were invited by Walt Disney Company CEO Bob Iger to join him in the Magic Kingdom for the dedication of a plaque honoring Randy. Standing in front of the topiaries by the Alice in Wonderland teacup ride, the children cut the ribbon around a leaf-shaped plaque with several quotes from Randy. It read: "Be good at something; it makes you valuable. . . . Have something to bring to the table because that will make you more welcome." After studying the plaque for a few minutes, Dylan asked Mr. Iger why Disney had chosen the shape of a leaf; he answered that the leaf symbolized their father's evergreen legacy, living on forever. What a unique opportunity for Dylan to have a conversation with the chief executive officer of one of the most influential companies in the world! After the ceremony, the children and I enjoyed the park with Randy's mother, his sister and her family, my brother and his daughter. It was a mini family reunion.

Later that same year, we were invited to Pittsburgh for the Randy Pausch Memorial Bridge dedication. Once again, the children did the honors at the ribbon-cutting ceremony to open the bridge that connects the Purnell Center for the Arts with the new Gates Center for Computer Science and the Hillman Center for Future-Generation Technologies, the latter two being the new home for computer science at Carnegie Mellon University. Without any trepidation whatsoever, Logan and Chloe spoke into the microphone to thank Carnegie Mellon for honoring their father. Dylan followed his siblings' example and made a comparison between the bridge lighting up the night and his father alight with life. The children then ran back and forth on the bridge as the seven thousand programmable LED lights created a light show that moved down it. The whole experience was made even more special because Randy's mother, sister, niece, and nephew were there with us. The next morning we walked over to a great little restaurant and had breakfast together. It reminded me of the times Randy and I would travel to his parents' house to meet his family and we would spend the weekend together.

The children have also traveled with me to Washington, D.C., where we participated in a walk to raise funds and awareness for pancreatic cancer research. Dylan and Logan were invited to give the kickoff address to the crowd of two thousand participants, which included their grandmother, aunt, and cousins. Neither one of them was intimidated to look out into the crowd and speak into the microphone. I was very impressed by their confidence and presence of mind to be able to talk about pancreatic cancer and its impact on them personally.

The following day, Dylan and I went to Capitol Hill to meet with Speaker of the House Nancy Pelosi, Representative Frank Pallone Jr., Senator Mark Warner, Representative Lucille Roybal-Allard, Senator Jim Webb, Representative Rosa DeLauro, and Representative J. Randy Forbes to ask for their support to increase funding for the National Cancer Institute and for pancreatic cancer research in particular. It was an incredible lesson for a child to learn—that as Americans we can go to our elected officials and talk with them about the issues we are concerned about and bring them to our government's attention. This was government "by the people, for the people," as Abraham Lincoln so famously put it in his Gettysburg Address. Furthermore, we were a part of a larger community of people affected by pancreatic cancer. Every year over 43,000 people nationwide are diagnosed with pancreatic cancer. Over 400 people from forty-nine states came together for this event. Dylan, Logan, and Chloe met other children who had lost a parent, a grandparent, or other loved one to the disease, which helped them see that they are not the only ones who have endured such a tragedy. They also met many people who were survivors, which gave all of us hope that one day more than 6 percent of those diagnosed with pancreatic cancer would be alive five years later. It was an incredible trip and one I hope we are able to repeat in the future.

Almost a year after I lost my engagement ring, I was cleaning out the purse I had used on our trip to the water park when, lo and behold, I discovered the ring in the center zipper compartment. How in the world it got there I will never know. I searched that purse right after I discovered the ring was missing. It is also not my habit to put jewelry in my purse when I leave a hotel room; I put it in the hotel room safe, with my watch and other valuables. In all the months I used that purse after the water park adventure, I never came across the ring. I was absolutely baffled but utterly euphoric to have it back. It resurfaced at a very interesting time in my life; I had decided to get back into the dating world. Maybe Randy returned the ring to me as a reminder of him and our relationship to help guide me as I searched my heart to see if it had healed enough to love again.

18

To Date or Not to Date

ONE OF THE MOST AWKWARD conversations I had with Randy as we prepared for his death dealt with the question of my remarrying. In his usual up-front manner, Randy counseled me on finding the right man and warned me to avoid the mistakes of my youth. He was so worried for me and for his children, who would be directly affected by whomever I chose to share my life with. I know I would have felt the same way if the shoe had been on the other foot and I had to trust Randy to find not only someone he loved and respected, but also someone who would be a great mother to my children. He also anticipated the public's curiosity about how he felt about the matter of my moving on romantically after he died, and he addressed this in *The Last Lecture*. "Most of all, I want Jai to be happy in the years ahead. So if she finds happiness through remarriage, that will be great. If she finds happiness without remarrying, that will also be great." He nicely worded

this phrase so that I wouldn't feel pressure to remarry, but I knew
how he was hedging his bets.

Before Randy died, he composed a short list of available men
whom he trusted and recommended that I consider them for courtship and possibly for marriage. Some of the folks I've told this story
to have reacted with indignation at how controlling Randy was in
his attempt to reach beyond the grave to manipulate my life. I don't
see it that way at all. Instead, I see a man who loved me so much that
he was able to put aside all jealousy at the thought of my being with
someone else and think about my happiness and the well-being of
our children. But I made him stop showing me the list, and I refused
to talk about other men with him when he pressed the subject on
me. I wasn't in an emotional space to consider the romantic aspect
of my future or the lack thereof.

After Randy had passed away, I was visiting with some of our
friends from church when my girlfriend told me about a conversation Randy had had with her and her husband. He asked our friends
to keep a lookout for a nice guy for me when the time was right.
Not only had Randy been keeping a list, but he had also enlisted
some of our friends to take on the role of my personal matchmaker!
Still, I wasn't ready to take that step and I thanked her for being
such a good friend.

I remember talking to Dr. Reiss in the fall of 2008, admitting
that I couldn't imagine being romantic with anyone at that moment
because I couldn't entertain the thought of opening up my heart or
risk getting hurt again. I was still overwhelmed with pain; my heart
wasn't up to the challenge of dating. My family watched over me
and silently waited until I was ready to venture back into the world
of romance, never pushing me to go where I wasn't ready. Later
on, I would learn how difficult it was for them as I mourned and

remained alone night after night, month after month. I had a wound that would heal according to no specific time line.

Randy's mother and sister were supportive of me on the issue of moving on romantically, though I don't believe Randy had asked them to assist me in this endeavor. Tammy, Randy's sister, and Virginia, his mother, are reasonable and loving people who understood that I might want to find someone someday to love again. One weekend when Tammy was visiting us, after the children were in bed, she brought up the topic of dating with me. She reassured me that she did not have a problem with my dating and wanted me to feel comfortable talking with her about the subject. It was wonderful to me that she broached the subject—one I had felt too uncomfortable to mention. It also made me feel closer to Randy's family, knowing that even difficult subjects such as dating and remarriage weren't going to be land mines in our relationship.

Oddly enough, the people who turned out to be the most vocal proponents for dating were my children, especially my oldest son, Dylan, who was seven at the time. I remember him talking to me about the subject one morning in the car after we had dropped off his siblings at preschool. He asked me if I would ever get remarried or if I had thought about the idea. I was completely caught off guard, not having had any dates or even talked about dating at this point. It must have been something he had given quite a bit of thought to, because he was prepared to have the discussion. So I tried to explain that Mommy wasn't ready yet because her heart still hurt after losing Daddy. I added that it would be difficult for Mommy to meet people, given my lack of social opportunities, and that he should understand it would be a while before I ventured into the dating world. Then my precocious son offered some strategies to help his forty-two-year-old mom meet an eligible man. "Have you thought about a divorced man? Because he might be looking for a new family," Dylan advised. Wow! Was I surprised by his reasoning and perception.

Later on, in another conversation, Dylan told me he missed his father and really wanted another dad. He was looking to me to find him another father to fill the void Randy left. Nothing like a little pressure from your child! Nothing like raising the ante when the stakes were already so high!

I told him how sorry I was that his father had died. I pointed out how lucky we were to have Uncle Bob, my brother, close by to come over and visit. And that many, many people loved us and helped us. These people didn't replace Randy, Dylan's father and best friend, but their presence was something we should appreciate. The truth is, I didn't want to go out into the dating world with the objective of giving my children another father. I don't think that's right, and I don't think it's fair. Bringing another man into this family isn't going to make our hurt go away or those feelings of missing Randy disappear. That was the real issue I wanted to address with Dylan—that it was OK to miss Randy, to miss having a dad, but he should not believe that substituting another person in Randy's place would make everything better. It was such a tough lesson for so young a person to have to learn, but very important.

By the summer of 2009, I was dealing much better with grief and life as a single parent. The knot in my chest had loosened, though not gone away completely. I felt comfortable with our daily routine. The kids were doing well and enjoying themselves. I loved watching them grow, sharing the day with them, and hatching new adventures. I also was developing a social network outside my immediate family. My friends and I would go out on occasion for dinner, to a movie, or to the theatre. Overall, I was feeling happy with my life. I wasn't alone, but I was starting to feel lonely. I missed holding someone's hand or snuggling while watching a movie. My heart was starting to thump again, and I was slowly becoming aware of its beating. It's not as though I woke up one morning and said, "Gee, I'd like to have someone special in my life starting today." Rather, it was a gradual awakening.

By the fall of 2009, a little over a year after Randy's death, I had given a few talks about my caregiving experience and about widowhood to a few health agencies and at a couple of pancreatic cancer fund-raisers. At each event, I would talk about Randy and our experiences together during his illness. But in talking about him and sharing my feelings about him with the audience, I felt I was conjuring his ghost, resurrecting him in such a way that I could feel him close to me again. It's interesting that I couldn't really talk about Randy or our experiences with our friends because it was too painful for everyone involved. Here in this public but also anonymous venue, it was not only OK for me to say his name and speak about the agonies cancer created in our lives, but the people attending these events wanted to know about them. They were eager to hear the details of our cancer journey, and I wanted to describe the pain cancer had caused for me, my husband, and our children. It was a cathartic, wonderful healing process. But as soon as the talk was over or I had left the fund-raiser, Randy's ghost would dissipate, and the feeling that he was with me would evaporate as well. I would lose him all over again.

And then loneliness would well up inside me. I didn't have that special person anymore with whom to share life's little joys. I loved Randy, I still do, but I decided I couldn't be married to a ghost. I needed more. I was content with my life, had wonderful friends, a close family who was very supportive, and new ventures that challenged me intellectually. I could go on like this, and it would be fine. But I want more than fine.

I decided I was ready to take another step forward in the direction of building my new life, but the decision presented me with a challenge: how to go about meeting someone. I met Randy when I was working. I had met the other men I'd dated, before marrying Randy, when I was a student taking classes. However, now I was neither in an office nor on a college campus. Bars were never my thing, so that option was out. It's no surprise that I didn't meet a guy playing women's tennis or picking up children at preschool or at elementary school functions. Nor did I meet anyone at church. When I started feeling exasperated, I turned to my friends and family for help. This method had worked brilliantly when I was looking for a pediatrician for the kids, a general practitioner for myself, a painter for the house, and a dog for the family. Surely my friends would be able to suggest an acceptable single man who would work out just as well as my electrician. How naive of me to think it would be so simple to find someone my age who was eligible to go out for dinner.

After a while, I got tired of hearing myself complain about the lack of progress in my romantic endeavors. The situation was becoming a real challenge and one I was determined to solve. I had to think out of the box and move to a less traditional dating method, since what I had been trying wasn't successful. And so, like 20 million other Americans, I signed up with an online dating service to increase my chances of meeting someone single. Twenty-four hours after I had enrolled, my account showed a list of at least ten eligible bachelors in my area. I was surprised by how easy and quick it was to have a list of potential dates within such a short period of time. It made me feel I had options. Let me clarify that statement. It wasn't that the online site provided me with a variety of men to choose from, but rather that it gave me the opportunity to meet single men or choose not to meet anyone. I wasn't forced by circumstance to be single; I had a choice, and that was so empowering to me.

Now that I actually had the chance to meet someone new, I had to make sure I was completely OK with moving on. In my heart, I knew I would always love Randy. In my mind, I recognized that our marriage vows released me from our bonds of matrimony when Randy died. Still, I had to wrestle a little bit with the feeling that I was cheating on my dead husband. My friends and counselor were there to listen to me and give me the support I needed to move forward with my life. They cautioned me to take things slowly, not to give my heart away too quickly, and most of all, just to have fun. So I took a deep breath and responded to the messages in my online dating account.

Dating in the abstract sounds very exciting, but in reality, it's difficult and painful. Rejection isn't something anyone enjoys at any age or stage of life, but it's part of dating. Of course, the upside is the surge of emotions one gets while getting to know someone new. It had been a long time since I had felt like this, and it was nice. Dating added a new and enriching dimension to my life, separate from my children and their lives and completely separate from my history with Randy—or so I thought.

I was surprised to find that my name and my face were recognizable even though more than a year had gone by since *The Last Lecture* had been published and any news about me had been aired. My hair had grown longer, and I felt I looked very different from the pictures of me that had been posted on the Internet, used on television, or printed in the book. Sometimes in an attempt to be candid, I would be very up-front about who my late husband was. Some potential dates have googled my name and learned a lot about me from the Internet. Both scenarios, I realized, created an imbalance of information between myself and the person I was getting to know. They knew a lot about me—how I met my husband, the births of our children, and how my marriage ended. I, on the other hand, knew little about them and felt at a disadvantage. I had to rely only on these men telling me the truth about themselves and how and why they were no longer married. And the public perception of Randy as a perfect person, even though he had his flaws, can be very intimidating to some men. Sometimes people can't help but see me as the professor's widow, and it can be quite off-putting. Randy's ghost seemed to haunt me when I was trying to move forward. I had to learn to handle these scenarios and get comfortable with who I was. Easier said than done.

Another complicating factor in dating is having small children. Because of their vulnerability, I want to protect them from getting attached to someone who might not be in our lives long-term. When I first started dating, I told the children I was going out to dinner with a man. Instantly they jumped to the conclusion that my date and I were getting married and they would finally have another dad. I explained to them that dating was a long process of getting to know someone before you made the decision to spend your life with that person. I shared Randy's mantra, "Marry in haste, repent at leisure," which led to a great discussion about the important attributes of a relationship worthy of matrimony. It's a great lesson for the children to learn and a silver lining to my widowhood. Logan gets very engaged in these discussions; he had developed an eye for the ladies at the tender age of five. I hope our discussions will help him make good choices when he gets to the point of going out with girls. My actions will also be an example for Chloe, which weighs on my mind as well. I want my daughter to see me with someone who treats me with love and kindness so that she will hold out for the same when she takes an interest in young men. How much easier it was to date when I was in college and worried only about how handsome a boy was!

Furthermore, I've had to learn *when* to introduce a person I'm seeing to my children. I don't want them to meet someone I'm not serious about or who isn't serious about me and my family. I don't want them to get emotionally attached to someone who might be around for only a few weeks. There's also the time necessary for me to develop a relationship with someone separate from and outside the spectrum of my family circle, time to learn about each other and grow into our relationship. I've had difficulty creating opportunities for the person I'm dating to spend time my children because of my desire to protect my kids. I know it's important for me to see how a man interacts with my children and vice versa. When I was talking about this very subject with Dylan, he came up with a metric of fifteen dates for me to use as a gauge for when it would be appropriate for me to bring somebody home to meet him and his siblings! I don't know if that's the best measuring stick, but I'm really glad I can talk with Dylan, Logan, and Chloe about this issue.

Dating takes a lot of time and energy. When I last dated, I had only myself to think about. Now I have to balance time with a man I'm dating against time with my children, who are my first priority. When I first started to go out again, I immediately wanted to stop, for fear that it would detract from other projects and from raising my children. One of my greatest passions right now has been to continue Randy's efforts to increase awareness and funding for pancreatic cancer research. I had always planned to volunteer in the cancer world in some way. I didn't realize that my dream underestimated what was really possible.

19

—⟨⟨⟨⟩⟩⟩—

Giving Back—
Pancreatic Cancer Advocate

ANDY AND I OFTEN WENT to an oncology appointment expecting to be in the cancer facility for three hours, only to find ourselves still there after four, five, or six hours. There were many different reasons for the delays. Sometimes, the nurse would have to infuse the chemotherapy drugs at a slower rate so as not to overload Randy's system. Sometimes he might need a shot to boost his white blood cell count. And sometimes the infusion area was so full of patients that there wasn't a chair for him. We had to wait our turn, kind of like waiting for a table at a restaurant, except Randy and the other patients were guaranteed to get sick from whatever they were served.

Most oncology departments recognize the fluid nature of chemotherapy appointments and keep a selection of drinks and snacks or vending machines available for their patients as they wait. There are also volunteers who come around the waiting rooms offering drinks and a sandwich to either the patient or caregiver. I can't tell you how many times I had lunch courtesy of these kind souls. MD Anderson Center in Houston covers ten thousand acres and employs seventeen thousand people. When Randy was undergoing the clinical trial treatment there, we would often be very far from a cafeteria or vending machine. Luckily for us and the other twenty thousand patients receiving care there, volunteers go around to different departments and waiting rooms with the Jolly Trolley—a cart stocked with snacks and hot coffee, tea, or chocolate. I can still hear the sound of the trolley's bell. That tinkling sound was welcomed by the hordes of us stuck in the bowels of the cancer center maze, where no sunlight penetrated and time was measured by the drips from the IV bag down the line. Cancer takes over more than just the body; it takes over one's time, takes away control over one's schedule, one's day. The patient and caregiver are completely in cancer's grip. The Jolly Trolley was more than a hot cup of coffee; it was a nice diversion from the reality of the moment served up with a friendly smile.

After spending long days that added up to weeks inside the cancer bureaucracy, I knew I wanted to help other people who were going through similarly trying times. When routine was restored within our household after Randy had passed, I wanted to use some of my free time while the children were in school and preschool to be a volunteer who handed out drinks and sandwiches to those now sitting in those same waiting rooms where I had been sitting just a short while ago. I knew from firsthand experience the difference such a simple act could make in someone's day. Rather than wallowing in my own self-pity, I would benefit from helping others. There's an immediate reward in doing for others—the instant gratification of interacting with the person you are helping. It's a much more personal experience than merely writing a check and putting it in the mail.

I'm sure some folks would never want to step back into a cancer ward, to see the IV poles and chemo bags strung up like party balloons. Some party! The guests are definitely not having a good time. They're not vomiting into the garbage can because they've had too much to drink. These reminders of darker days reopen wounds for those of us who have survived a cancer experience. I know the pain of patients and caregivers, and I understand why some people do not volunteer in some way. The experience is devastating for everyone. For my part, I needed to do something to help the people who were still sitting in those wards, all suffering silently in their own ways. After seeing the atrocities cancer can do to body and spirit, I felt great empathy for those walking in my shoes. I couldn't shut out the images by closing my eyes; they would only reappear in my mind.

My volunteering plans took a turn, though, in the fall of 2008 when Julie Fleshman, president of the Pancreatic Cancer Action Network, called me and asked me to attend the organization's annual fund-raiser. A year later, she asked me to join the organization's board of directors. I hesitated because I wasn't sure I had the time or experience to give to the organization at this level. Still, I didn't say no right away but instead took a little time to talk it over with several close friends. My reservations included being newly widowed and dealing with a tsunami of grief, as well as learning to be a single parent. My lack of experience as a board member also gave me pause. The only experience I had was serving on the Pittsburgh Toy Lending Library's board, which was no comparison in terms of scope or budget to the Pancreatic Cancer Action Network. Then there was the fact that my free time was limited because Chloe was in preschool for only four hours a day. Serving on the Pancreatic Cancer Action Network's board would knock out my designs to serve as a refreshment volunteer. I couldn't do both, so I had to choose.

In the end, I decided this offer was an opportunity I didn't want to pass up. Maybe I wouldn't be doing something as tangible as handing out food, but I would be playing a similar role on a larger scale. I liked becoming part of a team whose goals aligned with mine. It would give me opportunities to meet other people affected by pancreatic cancer who wanted to do something about the disease. Even though there is only a 10 percent chance of inheriting pancreatic cancer, I didn't like to think about my children being afflicted with the disease that killed their father, especially when the survival rate hasn't changed in forty years. What hope would medical science have to offer to my children at this pace of discovery? How would I feel if I hadn't done all that I could to change the landscape of this disease?

As these ideas swirled around in my head, I thought about Randy. He never encouraged me to continue his crusade. His actions, though, spoke volumes. When he was in the hospital for congestive heart failure and kidney failure in March 2008, he told the doctors he needed to be released in time to go to Washington, D.C., to testify in front of Congress and advocate for greater funding for the National Cancer Institute and for pancreatic cancer. The doctors did release him, even though we were still trying to get his blood pressure down from 200/100. Randy was in a lot of discomfort, and he was very weak. Just watch the video of his testimony filmed by Geoff Martz of ABC News. You can see Randy grab his sides and grimace in pain. Nevertheless, he willed himself to get dressed and suffer the four-hour drive, resting in the back of the car.

Back in August 2007, Randy's doctors told him he would most likely not be alive after six months—in other words in March 2008. He told Diane Sawyer during an interview for an hour-long *20/20* television special in April 2008 that he didn't expect to be alive on Father's Day in June. He knew he was living on borrowed time. His decision to take another day away from his children after just having spent five days in the hospital where he didn't see them at all underscores how important it was to him to try to make a difference. Moreover, Randy knew that his efforts would not benefit himself in the least—it was too late for that. He went anyway, and I think he hoped not only to bring attention to pancreatic cancer, but to rally the public and our government to action—to get behind the medical researchers and give them the tools they need to find a cure. Short of this goal, he hoped to inspire others to pick up the baton and run the race that he couldn't finish. In a public service announcement he made, Randy said, "In all likelihood, cancer is going to defeat my body, but it's not going to defeat my soul because the human spirit is much more powerful than any biological disease." In light of his actions and words, how could I not pick up the baton and carry on in that spirit?

I accepted the Pancreatic Cancer Action Network's offer to join their board of directors. It is a decision I have not regretted. Because the organization has a comprehensive approach to attacking the disease, I have learned a lot—from the business of running a nonprofit to the art of marshaling volunteers. Being on the board doesn't mean sitting around a conference table looking at a stack of reports. Board members are active at the grassroots level. I have participated in organized community walks, raising awareness about the disease among the general public as well as raising funding. I've tried to include my children at events or activities when it's been appropriate, so we can be together as a family and learn through example and action what it means to give back to our community.

In addition to community events, I've done a lot of public speaking. These invitations have challenged me to develop a skill set that I didn't have before joining the Pancreatic Cancer Action Network. Before the birth of the children, I'd been a webmaster; I never set foot on a stage or picked up a microphone. As a graduate student at the University of North Carolina, I was nervous when I had to present a paper to my classmates and professor—about fifteen people. Now I walk onto a stage and address two thousand people but don't experience stage fright. My friends have asked me how I can stand in front of such a large group of people and keep my composure. It's because I really believe in what I'm doing. I have complete conviction that we as a society need to do more to help scientists make headway against this difficult and deadly disease. What Randy and I experienced was horrendous to both of us and to our families in ways that were unprecedented for us all. Talking about it helps me move forward. I hope that sharing my experience will cause others to identify with us and not feel so isolated going through their own journeys, and that they will in turn help my cause. I feel that some good has to come from the painful experience of Randy's battle with cancer and from our loss. This is the true silver lining—helping others while helping myself.

The more challenging aspect has been the business side of the nonprofit organization. As a board member, I am charged with ensuring the fiscal responsibility of the Pancreatic Cancer Action Network, which translates into making sure that any and all monies donated to the organization go toward its mission—curing pancreatic cancer. Luckily for me, the organization's accounting is transparent and well documented, making my job so much easier.

It's been a real eye-opener to see how a well-managed nonprofit is always trying to keep costs down and use its funds to the best advantage toward its goals. The position has made me think in ways I've never had to do before.

As I have continued my involvement in the pancreatic cancer community, I've had the privilege of meeting some super people working tirelessly to bring about a cure. One in particular who stands out as a role model for me is Roger Magowitz. I met Roger at a Pancreatic Cancer Action Network gala fund-raiser in October 2008. He offered me his business card and told me to call him if I ever needed a mattress (which I did!). At the time, Roger owned twenty mattress stores in Arizona and fifteen in Virginia. He and his wife, Jeanne, live not far from me in Virginia Beach, and we've become friends. I didn't know it at the time, but Roger had added me to his immense list of friends and contacts. Roger is a people maven, fitting Malcolm Gladwell's definition to a T. He has a vast network of friends through which he meets others or can get to know someone outside his own network through various degrees of separation. Roger uses his talent to help bring about a cure for pancreatic cancer because the disease took his own mother eight years earlier. Instead of remaining bitter, Roger channeled his energies and emotions into a full frontal assault on the disease. First, he volunteered to help organize a golf tournament to raise funds for the Pancreatic Cancer Action Network, which netted $10,000. The following year, he suggested to the organizer that the tournament be named after his mother, Seena Magowitz. Through his efforts and networking, the tournament raised $50,000 that year! When the organizer wanted to change the tournament's name each year to honor a different person, Roger knew his friends wouldn't come out as they had before, so he decided to go off on his own and start his own golf fund-raiser in his mother's honor. His network of friends and supporters followed him. The golf classic has grown both in the number of attendees (four hundred in 2010) and in dollars ($2.5 million in 2010). I am amazed at his success and determination, born of a desire to extinguish the disease that devastated his family when it took his mother's life.

The golf tournament isn't the only project Roger has undertaken in his quest to help conquer pancreatic cancer. He has galvanized his industry to implement some creative ideas. Roger initiated the novel idea of making teddy bears out of Tempur-Pedic's space-age foam and donating the proceeds to the Pancreatic Cancer Action Network. He also committed to purchase a percentage of the bears for his stores in Virginia. Roger's idea helped launch the "Hugs Back" campaign, in which Tempur-Pedic used those squeezable, huggable bears to raise awareness about pancreatic cancer through its marketing, advertising, and public relations. The company advertised the bears and the cause they represented in national and local magazines and newspaper print ads, along with television and radio spots, selling the bears for a modest amount at bedding stores across the country. By the end of December 2010, Tempur-Pedic's campaign had generated $300,000 for pancreatic cancer research, all because Roger challenged the bedding industry to care, and these corporate giants rose to the challenge.

When I talked to him about how he was able to manage a company in two different states while still volunteering his time to pancreatic cancer projects, Roger explained that he had been in the business for more than twenty years with an excellent staff in place to help to keep his business running. He never lost sight of the fact that his mother had died without hope of treatment or cure, and he was willing to put in 110 percent every day. When his friends and colleagues saw what he gave of his time, money, and resources to this cause, they were more willing to get involved. When Roger decided to sell his company, he chose a buyer that agreed to make pancreatic cancer research funding its corporate charity. Mattress Firm not only bought Roger's company; they also hired him to keep doing what he had already been doing all these years without compensation—fight pancreatic cancer. Moreover, Roger and his wife, Jeanne, pledged $1 million to the Translational Genomics Research Institute's physician-in-chief, Dr. Daniel Von Hoff, to underwrite his clinical trials so that treatment options make it from the medical research lab to the patient much faster. They could have chosen to buy a retirement home in Florida and play golf every day, and felt they had done their part. Instead, they led by example and tangibly showed that ending pancreatic cancer and helping others was a priority in their lives.

Because of people like Roger and Jeanne, I'm beginning to make choices about what is important to me and my family. I've had to ask myself how I want to handle the experience I went through with Randy. Do I want to bury it deep inside me and let time slowly repair that wound, or do I want to embrace my tragedy and use it to make something positive? At the same time, I don't want to be handcuffed to the past or defined by it. The next challenge I face is to learn how to take my experiences from the past and use them to make a difference in the world today without letting the past dictate my future. I don't want to be "Randy's widow," but just Jai Pausch. Somehow I must find a way to take the broken pieces of my dreams from yesterday and use them to create something new and beautiful that fits who I am today.

20

⁂

Dreaming New Dreams

ECENTLY I WAS ASKED to introduce Roger Magowitz at a Translational Genomics Research Institute founders dinner. I was looking forward to telling the guests about Roger's efforts and about the innovative work he helps fund: the pancreatic cancer research led by Dr. Daniel Von Hoff at TGen. As I looked around the room, my eyes fell upon a familiar face. *Where do I know him from?* I asked myself as I went through my talk. Then it dawned on me! That face belonged to Dan Quayle. Here was a former vice president of the United States sitting at the table just to my right, looking up at me and listening to what I had to say. Never in a million years would I ever have imagined myself in a position to have a vice president, former or present, listen attentively to me. What an incredible night that was. Later on, I thought about what I had experienced and what it meant. My take-home message is that even though I may not know what my future holds, I should not give in to the fear of the unknown. I have to trust. I have to have faith that my life will continue to have exciting and magical times. I just have to keep myself open to the possibilities.

Starting over is something we all do at various times throughout our lives for many different reasons, like divorcing or losing a job. Closing a chapter in life naturally creates fear and anxiety. In an interview with *O* magazine, Oprah Winfrey spoke very candidly about starting a new phase in her life after ending *The Oprah Winfrey Show*. Winfrey describes her pep talk to herself like this: "*Here you are, in bed, afraid of making the next move and look at where you are* [in her Maui home overlooking the water]. . . . *Look at where you have been brought from.* I started thinking about my little house in Mississippi, and I started to cry. I thought, *Look at all the times when God didn't leave you alone.* And I thought, *Okay, okay: God is not going to give me this opportunity and just leave me alone—why would I be put in this position, just to fail?*" Oprah didn't remain chained to her successful show, nor did she let anxiety about the future paralyze her from taking the next step. She owned that fear, harnessed its energy, and used it to create a new dream: a network dedicated to her own television programming.

I'm also beginning a new phase of my life and choosing not to be trapped by my past. I need to reinvent myself, adapt to the new circumstances I find myself in, and most important, grow. One of the greatest life lessons I've learned has been to dream new dreams. When a dream is fulfilled, it shouldn't become a straitjacket, constricting a person's evolution and progress. Instead, it should be a stepping-stone to the next thing. When a dream shatters, you should pick up the pieces and create a new one. It won't be the same as the broken one, but you can hope it will be as vibrant and as exciting. I've had to give myself permission to let go of old dreams—I'm not going to raise my children with the man I married on May 20, 2000, under the shade of two giant oak trees. That dream died with Randy, and now the shards lie about my feet. Nor can I continue to be tied to that moment in my life. What good would it do for Randy or my children if I stayed a grieving widow? What kind of example would I be for my children? Isn't it so much more healthy to move forward with the lessons I've learned, to heal my wounds and to continue to live my life? I remind myself of today's possibilities instead of yesterday's disappointments. I've created a new mantra: Dream new dreams.

Looking at the pieces of my old dream, I've tried to figure out how to salvage what I can to build a new vision. After much soul-searching and many deep breaths, I've taken stock of the positive opportunities in my life and begun to take small steps on the road to finding an appropriate direction for myself as well as my family. Those steps include nurturing my children, developing a network of friends, and opening up my heart again in the search for love. Recently, I've met a wonderful man, Rich Essenmacher, who accepts and loves me as well as Dylan, Logan, and Chloe. To be with someone whom I treasure and love is such a rare gift, one I can truly appreciate after the experiences I have had. After having to be strong for so long, I didn't realize how tiring the burden had become. Not until Rich took some of the load from my shoulders did I feel a sense of relief. Day by day, I learn to lean on him more, though I've had difficulty in allowing Rich to do things for me—simple things, like opening my car door. I didn't think my heart could beat so strongly again, but it has, and I am so glad.

Moving forward with a new love has forced me to reexamine how I spend my time. I acknowledge the importance of helping others. I continue to offer support and be a resource for widows and widowers who have lost their spouses to some form of cancer.

I also write an online column, *Ask Jai,* on the National Comprehensive Cancer Network website, offering advice to caregivers going through the cancer experience. By doing so, I feel I'm repaying some of the debt I owe for all the support I received over the past several years.

I feel so much positive energy in continuing to help the pancreatic cancer community. In addition to the Pancreatic Cancer Action Network, I joined forces with the Lustgarten Foundation and the Translational Genomics Research Institute to further promote education and research for pancreatic cancer. I give talks at cancer conferences and community centers to bring awareness to the plight of the caregiver, who often goes without support. I didn't seek out this role, but when the opportunity arose, I carefully evaluated it and decided that it was right for me. I would never have envisioned being a caregiver or a pancreatic cancer spokesperson. Though I want to continue to be a part of the cancer community, I know my energies and my time are limited. There is so much to be done.

I couldn't have thought about these opportunities or roles when I was young because I hadn't had these life experiences yet. You don't ever know in childhood or upon high school or college graduation what the future holds for you, what your greatest challenges or achievements will be. When former President Jimmy Carter was asked if he knew what he was going to be when he was a child growing up in rural Georgia on his father's peanut farm, he replied, "At that time, all I had as an ambition since I was five years old was to go to Annapolis and be a naval officer. I had a favorite uncle who was a sailor and he sent me mementos from the Philippines and Japan and China, so I wanted to be in the Navy. That was my only ambition, to be in the Navy." Look what Mr. Carter went on to do after he achieved his childhood dream of joining the Navy: thirty-ninth president of the United States and winner of the 2002 Nobel Peace Prize.

Childhood dreams, college dreams—they are just the beginning. They take you down a path that will bring many possibilities and directions from which to choose. The mistake we sometimes make is that we stop dreaming as we grow older, making it more difficult to cope with and recover from changes as they occur in life, when things don't go according to plan. Even when you find fulfillment, don't stop dreaming. Use that success to segue into the next phase of life.

As I write this, I have been a single parent for several years— several long, hard years, during which the children have grown both emotionally and physically. There have been many adjustments we've had to make individually and as a family. Happily, my children have shown resilience in their ability to accept our circumstances and to thrive.

The time we spend together as a family is invaluable, and I don't want anything I do to impinge on it. The children have been very receptive to my fiancé, who showers them with time and attention. Rich has shown me that he loves children, that he's willing to parent with me. It is all upside for my children, who remain my primary focus. Still, we are transitioning into a blended family, learning about each other and how to live together harmoniously. Patience, time, and love will make all the difference in creating the glue that will bond us together.

We maintain very close family relationships, sharing our thoughts and feelings. I've also tried to continue to instill the values that Randy and I cherished. Pitching in around the house is important, both for me as a single parent and for the children to learn about responsibility. They work together as a team, loading and unloading the dishwasher, taking out the trash and recycling, helping to clean out the car, keeping their rooms and toys organized, and putting away their clothes. They're proud of their work and taking an active role in the household. They know their efforts make a difference for me and for us. I couldn't be prouder of the bond we've forged together.

I'm also amazed at each child's individual growth. Our oldest son, Dylan, is now ten and a half years old and is a fourth grader. He's making friends at school and progressing nicely in academics. He continues to remind me of his father in his way of speaking, his ability to grasp complex subjects, his natural ability to negotiate, and his empathy. Dylan surprises me in many ways, and I love watching him grow up. Often he catches me by surprise when he makes a statement that is wise beyond his years. When Dylan talks, I hear his father—the way his brain worked and processed the world around him.

At seven and a half, Logan's laughter and love of life are as spirited as ever. With his impish smile and curly brown hair, he wins friends easily. More important, he has a kind heart and is loyal to his family and friends. Like his father, he loves computers and gadgets. When the children want to watch a DVD, play a computer game, or troubleshoot one of their electronic devices, they go see Logan, who tinkers around until he fixes the problem. He is also athletic and uses his considerable strength when he plays soccer or wrestles with his brother. What I love best about Logan is his willingness to show his love for you with a hug or by snuggling on the couch.

At six, Chloe has demonstrated an amazing attitude of independence and persistence. For six months when she was four, she asked to buzz-cut her hair to look like her brothers, even after I explained that she would look different from the other girls and might experience some teasing. Still, my strong-willed daughter had made up her mind and knew what she wanted. After the locks were shorn off, Chloe looked beautiful, and she danced around happy and excited. Later on, she learned what peer pressure feels like and has since decided to grow her hair out. I'm so glad she had this experience in a loving and supportive environment. As I told her repeatedly, I would love her with or without hair, because it's not what she looks like on the outside, but rather who she is on the inside. She is a joy to have in my life.

As much as I love my children, it pains me greatly when they are sad and missing their father. When Dylan, Logan, and Chloe express their sadness, I try to soothe them and hold them until the waves of grief pass. Making time for them and listening to them helps them feel comfortable in talking about their sorrow and not keeping it bottled up. While I can't mend their broken hearts, I can let them know I'm here for them and that I love them. Sometimes that's all you can do besides offering a hug.

I've also learned that children grieve differently than adults. My grief was greatest immediately after Randy's death; those intense feelings have slowly subsided. Though also powerful after Randy's passing, the children's grief seems to recur at different times, flaring up and then quieting down again. A developmental milestone or being overly tired can trigger their feelings, causing tears to stream down their little faces. Each time, I hold them and tell them it will get better and they won't always be this sad. I'm mindful that this process will continue throughout their young lives, as opposed to being over and done within a certain period. Having a good foundation for handling their sorrow will be an important asset as they grow up. In order to create that, I need to be on hand for them here, right now.

We are truly blessed in that I don't have to go back to work and can stay home with my children. I am very aware that this is not the case for many people, who struggle financially when they lose a spouse. I recognize this opportunity is a gift that shouldn't be squandered. As I think about what I want to do to develop my life, I keep in mind that their needs are first and foremost. That means I maintain a healthy balance between my children's needs and my own. I continue to support pancreatic cancer education and research and to foster awareness about the needs of caregivers, but I carefully select my activities outside the home so as to minimize the impact on my time with my family. This is something completely new to me, since I have always been a stay-at-home mother and haven't been in a situation of having to turn down requests. Learning to say no is a new life lesson but essential so as not to take on too many projects. I also limit my travel to once every two months to reduce my time away from my children. So far these strategies have worked well, and we have all reaped the rewards.

In pursuing my own path in life, I have met some incredible people and found myself in the most amazing situations. Although it has been exciting to meet famous people, the really meaningful moments have come from seeing the difference my efforts have made in other people's lives. It is then that I can feel my energies are not in vain, that this is the right thing for me to be doing—at least for now. By remaining mindful of my mantra, "Dream new dreams," I hope to continue to grow in directions that are meaningful to me, rather than become stagnant or in an unhappy routine. As life throws curveballs at me, I'll be able to evaluate how these new challenges affect my current situation and then make changes accordingly. If my activities become too much for me or my family,

I retain the flexibility to do things differently, either by cutting back or by finding a different channel for my energies and goals.

Not all my aspirations are pinned on cancer and caregiver issues. One of my long-term dreams has been to travel more. The desire comes naturally to me because my father was a marine and we moved every three years to different cities across the country. When my life was at its lowest point over these past several years, I would get through the tough times by thinking about visiting some foreign country. I could envision myself stepping onto the plane, relaxing in my seat, and feeling the plane lift off the ground. In my mind's eye, I created all sorts of adventures, from riding a camel and seeing the pyramids in Egypt to taking a bicycle tour of France's wine country. After my trip to Italy with my best friend, Tina Carr, I understood that I should not put off doing something for myself now, not delay it until later in my life. I need to derive some enjoyment from each day, not wait until tomorrow. Too many things can happen between now and then. Too many what-ifs could throw a wrench in my deferred gratification plan. Already I'm looking forward to my vacation this year, and I'm dreaming of some lovely, exciting journeys for the near future.

Life is a precious gift, and I don't intend to waste a day of it. Have I experienced tragedy? Yes, I have. But it would be another real tragedy if I didn't recover from the sadness I have felt and thus missed the many happy moments along the way. Was my dream crushed? Yes, it was. And that will happen again. But when it does, I will pick up those pieces and create something new. I will always dream new dreams.

RESOURCES

The Pancreatic Cancer Action Network
Pancreatic Cancer Action Network is the national organization creating hope in a comprehensive way through research, patient support, community outreach, an advocacy for a cure. The organization raises money for direct private funding of research—and advocates for more aggressive federal research funding of medical breakthroughs in prevention, diagnosis, and treatment of pancreatic cancer.
> www.pancan.org; info@pancan.org;
> www.facebook.com/JointheFight
> 1500 Rosecrans Avenue, Suite 200, Manhattan Beach, CA 90266
> 310-725-0025; toll free: 877-272-6226

The Lustgarten Foundation
The Lustgarten Foundation is America's largest private foundation dedicated solely to funding pancreatic cancer research. Because Cablevision Systems Corporation underwrites all of the Lustgarten Foundation's administrative costs, 100 percent of every dollar donated to the foundation goes directly to pancreatic cancer research.
> www.lustgarten.org; www.curePC.org;
> www.facebook.com/CurePancreaticCancer
> 1111 Stewart Avenue, Bethpage, NY 11714
> 516-803-2304; toll free: 1-866-1000; fax: 516-803-2303

Dr. Daniel Von Hoff and his team
The Translational Genomics Research Institute
TGen's mission is to rapidly develop new treatments and better diagnostics for pancreatic cancer and other deadly diseases.
> www.helptgen.org; foundation@gen.org; www.facebook.com/helptgen
> 445 N. Fifth Street, Phoenix, AZ 85004
> 602-343-8400; toll free 1-866-370-8436

The Seena Magowitz Foundation: The Face and Voice for Pancreatic Cancer
> www.seenamagowitzfoundation.org;
> www.facebook.com/pages/Seena-Magowitz-Foundation/275193745486
> Roger E. Magowitz, Founder and Chairman
> roger@seenamagowitzfoundation.org; 602-524-7636

ACKNOWLEDGMENTS

I would like to thank Dylan, Logan, and Chloe for their love which has inspired me to be the best person and mom I could be. You amaze me every day.

Thank you for agreeing to go out to dinner, Rich. I didn't know I could love so deeply again. With you I learned to open up my heart, let go of the past, and make a future for us.

There aren't enough words of gratitude for all my friends and family who pitched in to help my family survive every day and each unique crisis. Many thanks to the Carnegie Mellon community, the First Unitarian Universalist Church of Pittsburgh, the Pausch and Glasgow families, and the Great Bridge community of friends, including my tennis teammates. Your actions renewed my faith.

Bob and Jane Glasgow were a strong presence during this ordeal, giving so much of themselves. Even when asked to do the impossible, Bob tried. I'm sorry I had unrealistic expectations.

For the caregiver who needs help, I would recommend Dr. Michele Reiss's book, *Lessons in Loss and Living*. Available online for free is the Johns Hopkins caregiver video series called *Walking on Eggshells*, www.hopkinsmedicine.org/kimmel_cancer_center/patient _information/videos/caregivers.html. In addition, many cancer centers and oncology centers offer caregiver support groups and counseling.

For those who are facing pancreatic cancer, I wholeheartedly recommend the Pancreatic Cancer Action Network's free Patients and

Liaison Service Program, www.pancan.org; 877-272-6226. The National Comprehensive Cancer Network, www.nccn.org, produces a free online patient pancreatic cancer guideline (as well as for a host of other cancers) to help patients and loved ones understand the disease and learn what their options are.

I'd like to salute the following organizations, researchers, and their volunteers for their continued efforts to find a cure for pancreatic cancer and to offer hope to patients and their families:

The Pancreatic Cancer Action Network

The Lustgarten Foundation

Dr. Daniel Von Hoff and his team at the Translational Genomics Research Institute

The Seena Magowitz Foundation